COMMONSENSE CARDIOLOGY

Dr George Strube
Dr Gillian Strube
General Practitioners,
Crawley, Sussex

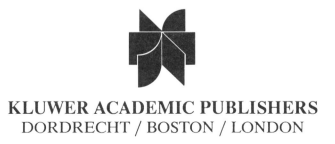

KLUWER ACADEMIC PUBLISHERS
DORDRECHT / BOSTON / LONDON

Distributors

for the United States and Canada: Kluwer Academic Publishers, PO Box 358, Accord Station, Hingham, MA 02018-0358, USA
for all other countries: Kluwer Academic Publishers Group, Distribution Center, PO Box 322, 3300 AH Dordrecht, The Netherlands

British Library Cataloguing in Publication Data

Strube, George
    Commonsense cardiology.
    1. Medicine. Cardiology
    I. Title   II. Strube, Gillian
    616.1´2

    ISBN 0-7462-0078-1

Library of Congress Cataloging in Publication Data

Strube, George.
    Commonsense cardiology / George Strube, Gillian Strube.
        p. cm.
    Includes index.
    ISBN 0-7462-0078-1 : £25.00 (U.K. : est.)
    1. Cardiology. 2. Heart – Diseases. I. Strube, Gillian.
II. Title.
    [DNLM: 1. Cardiology. 2. Heart – Diseases. WG 100 S927c]
    RC681.S894 1988
    616.1´2 – dc19
    DNLM/DLC
    for Library of Congress   88-13304
                                                                     CIP

Copyright

Published in the United Kingdom by Kluwer Academic Publishers, PO Box 55, Lancaster, UK.

Kluwer Academic Publishers BV incorporates the publishing programmes of D. Reidel, Martinus Nijhoff, Dr W. Junk and MTP Press.

Printed in Great Britain by Butler and Tanner Ltd., Frome and London

COMMONSENSE CARDIOLOGY

Presented to

DR HASSAN

with the compliments of

Melinda Betwistle.

your Upjohn Representative

As a service to medical education

Contents

Preface

Cardiology embraces a number of different conditions and disease processes. Cardiovascular disease is now responsible for most of the deaths of adults, especially premature deaths, in the developed world.

The development of effective preventive measures, new drugs and surgical techniques makes it increasingly important to recognise those at risk, to diagnose accurately those suffering from disease and to prescribe, monitor and refer appropriately.

This book is intended to focus attention on the opportunities which family practice provides for this and to look at the need for a change in emphasis in approaching the problems.

The book is in five parts. Part 1 is a reminder of some of the basic principles, which are essential if sensible cardiology is to be practised. Part 2 is about cardiac drugs, their use, effectiveness and risks. Part 3 looks at the diagnostic process; it comprises the history, examination, investigation and referral of patients, who might have cardiac disease and also the drugs which are most likely to be used. Part 4 is devoted to specific conditions. In Part 5, we look at the need for prevention and consider how it may be tackled in general practice.

This is not a comprehensive textbook of cardiology. It is not intended for students. It is hoped that it may be useful to experienced doctors, struggling to provide a sound, sensible service in an environment of ever expanding technology.

Acknowledgement

We would like to thank Dr Richard Vincent, Consultant Cardiologist at the Royal Sussex County Hospital, Brighton, for his help, advice and limitless patience, particularly in choosing and providing the ECGs. He has given us much support and encouragement and contributed greatly to any merit the book may have. He is in no way responsible for its deficiencies.

PART 1:
THE BASICS

1.1

Introduction

This is a review of some of the basic principles of the physiology of the heart and circulation; not as an end in itself but as a means of providing the tools needed to practise commonsense cardiology in general practice.

Why basics?

Knowledge about the cardiovascular system, the disease processes which affect it and their treatment, has increased so much during recent years that there now exists an enormous mass of information, which is apparently essential to everyday practice and yet which it is beyond most of us to retain for more than a few minutes at a time.

We believe that the key to this dilemma lies in an understanding of the physiology, pathophysiology and pharmacology which underlie both the disease processes themselves and the use of drugs and other treatments in their management. They form a common thread, a logical link, which allows us to keep to a reasonable minimum the quantity of facts we have to remember. Using this approach, makes it easier:

(1)   to make accurate and consistent diagnoses;

(2)   to understand and use, safely and effectively, the vast panoply of powerful and potentially dangerous drugs now available;

(3)   to make logical and appropriate use of investigations and the services of specialists;

(4)   to understand and apply new technology, including drugs, as it is developed.

It could be said that we need to know more about less: to deepen our understanding and not add to the facts we struggle to remember. This is the stuff of commonsense.

This part of *Commonsense Cardiology* contains nothing new to anyone who was even half awake as a medical student. It is simply revision. We make no apologies for this: it has always been important. It is now indispensible because of the extent of modern developments.

Part 1 contains the following chapters:

Chapter 1.2: Basic Anatomy – illustrated by diagrams;

Chapter 1.3: Physiological Models – these are models of the cardiovascular system, with explanations;

Chapter 1.4: Electrophysiology.

Throughout the book we will return to these to see how they are disturbed by disease processes and influenced by treatment.

1.2
Basic Anatomy

This short chapter is a simple presentation of the basic anatomy of the cardiovascular system. Figure 1.2A shows the circulation. Figure 1.2B shows the distribution of the blood in different vessels. Figure 1.2C shows the heart, Figure 1.2D shows the position of the heart in the chest and Figure 1.2E shows the coronary arteries.

This outline may seem over-simplified but it serves to remind us that the cardiovascular system is made up of a two-chambered pump with lengths of piping and perfusion networks between the chambers.

It also serves as a framework for the discussion of cardiac physiology which follows in the next chapter.

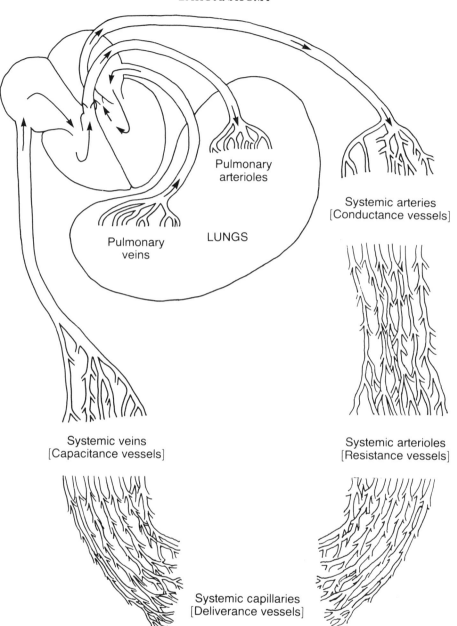

Pulmonary
arterioles

Systemic arteries
[Conductance vessels]

LUNGS

Pulmonary
veins

Systemic veins
[Capacitance vessels]

Systemic arterioles
[Resistance vessels]

Systemic capillaries
[Deliverance vessels]

Figure 1.2A Diagram of the circulation

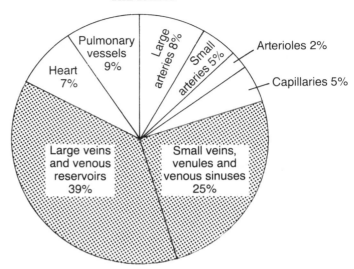

Figure 1.2B Distribution of the blood in different vessels

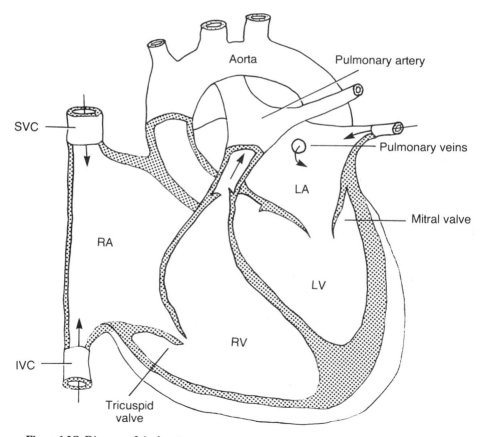

Figure 1.2C Diagram of the heart

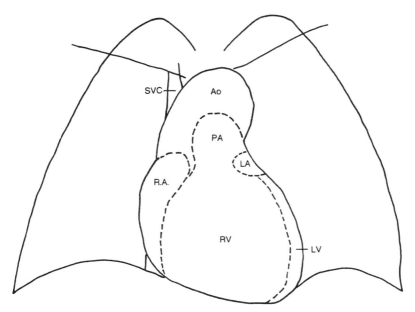

Figure 1.2D The heart is central. It does not normally occupy more than half of the diameter of the chest on an X-ray film (i.e. the cardiothoracic ration is less than 50%). The aortic and pulmonary valves are directly behind the sternum

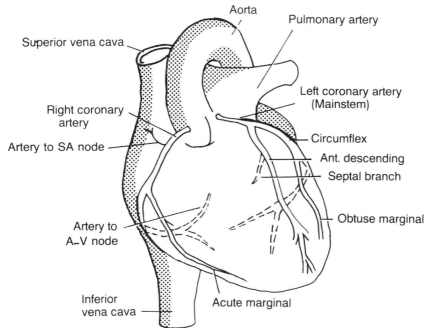

Figure 1.2E Diagram of coronary circulation: anterior view (arteries at the back are shown as dashed lines)

1.3
Physiological Models

THE BASIC MODEL

Figure 1.3A presents a basic model of cardiac physiology. Later models will expand on this with the addition of further detail.

The cardiovascular system is a closed system and except for very short periods, the output of the right side of the heart must be the same as that of the left. The two halves of the circulation have both similarities and differences. Two of the differences are especially important and have far-reaching effects: the pressures in the left side of the heart are far greater than those on the right and the capacity of the systemic peripheral vessels, especially the veins, is far greater than the capacity of those in the lungs.

These factors mean that the left ventricle has to work much harder than the right and is therefore more susceptible to strain and failure. When the left heart does fail, the back pressure into the lungs often has devastating effects. Pure right heart failure causes relatively few problems, unless it is severe, as its effects are absorbed by the peripheral vascular bed. The work of the heart can be reduced by diverting some of the circulating volume into the peripheral vascular bed and reducing the venous return to the right heart. This is what happens when a patient takes glyceryl trinitrate (GTN) for angina, or someone with acute left ventricular failure (LVF) sits on the edge of the bed with their legs hanging down.

Figure 1.3B is the same basic model with more detail. Much is self-evident but it is worth noting some of the relationships especially carefully.

There are separate links from heart rate to ventricular output and from heart rate to ventricular filling on each side.

These links are shown separately because heart rate affects cardiac output in two ways, which have opposite effects:

(1)   Ventricular output = stroke volume x heart rate, i.e. the more beats there are, the greater the output (as long as the stroke volume stays the same);

(2)   Stroke volume is inversely proportional to heart rate because the stroke volume, which is the amount the ventricle ejects during each contraction, depends on the amount of blood in the ventricle when it starts to contract.

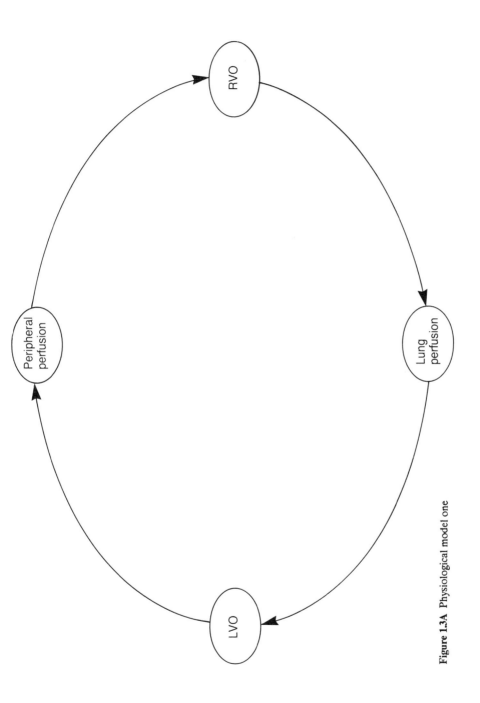

Figure 1.3A Physiological model one

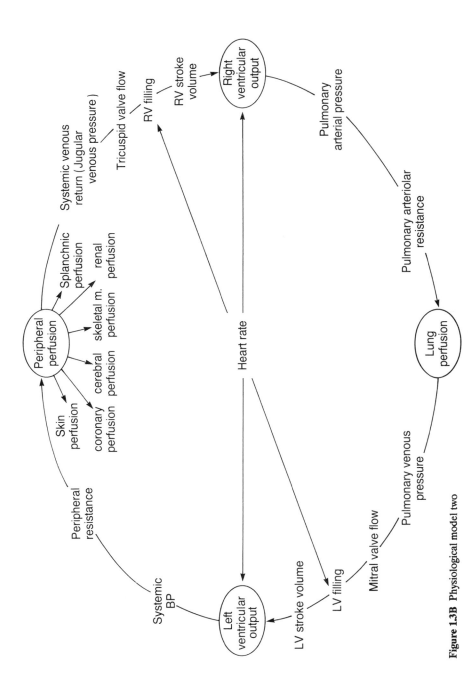

Figure 1.3B Physiological model two

This volume is the end diastolic volume (EDV) and it depends on the length of time the ventricle has had in which to fill (ventricular filling time). The ventricles fill during diastole.

The faster the heart rate, the shorter is diastole. In fact, diastole is shortened to a greater extent than systole, when the heart speeds up. Therefore, the faster the heart rate, the smaller the stroke volume.

Figures 1.3C and 1.3D show ventricular filling split into its two components: rate and time. The rate depends on the venous return to the heart and will be discussed later.

This explains why, although we all make use of a tachycardia to increase our cardiac output during exercise, an excessive tachycardia, as in atrial fibrillation, reduces cardiac output. On the other hand, a pathological bradycardia, while allowing plenty of time for the ventricles to fill, reduces the number of beats so much that overall output falls.

Peripheral resistance

Peripheral resistance depends on peripheral arteriolar tone. Peripheral resistance is also called systemic vascular resistance (SVR). It is the left ventricular output (LVO) working against the SVR which produces the systemic blood pressure (BP):

$$LVO \times SVR = BP$$

or, flow = pressure/resistance (Ohm's law)

If the SVR rises, the blood pressure rises, as long as the left ventricle can keep output the same. The blood pressure also rises if the cardiac output increases, but the peripheral resistance stays the same.

There are often changes in both parameters. For instance, during exercise the peripheral resistance falls, due to arteriolar dilatation and increased blood flow to skeletal muscles but the cardiac output rises so much that the blood pressure rises. This is such a consistent response that it can be used as a measure of left ventricular function. If, during an exercise test, the blood pressure fails to rise, this is taken as evidence of poor left ventricular function and is a poor prognostic sign.

Figure 1.3E (page 14) shows the pressures in different parts of the circulation.

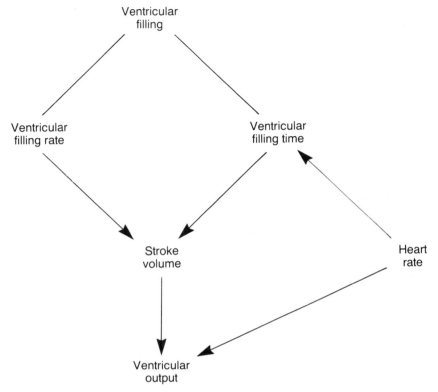

Figure 1.3C Relationship between SV, HR, filling time and CO.

    ventricular filling time $\propto \dfrac{1}{\text{heart rate}}$

∴   stroke volume $\propto \dfrac{1}{\text{heart rate}}$

∴   although ventricular output = stroke volume x heart rate, an increase in heart rate reduces stroke volume

∴   an increase in heart rate causes an increase in ventricular output only as long as the increased number of beats compensates for the reduced volume of each

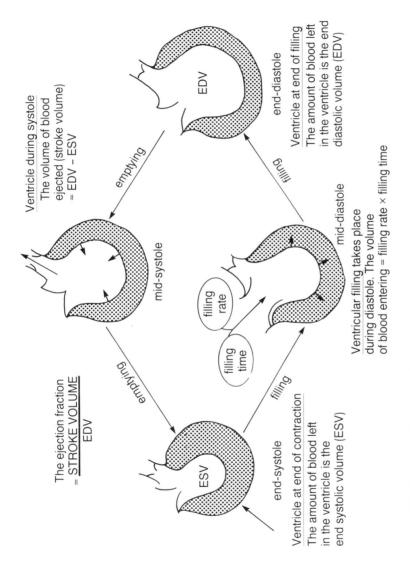

Ventricle during systole
The volume of blood
ejected (stroke volume)
= EDV − ESV

emptying

mid-systole

filling

end-diastole
Ventricle at end of filling
The amount of blood left
in the ventricle is the end
diastolic volume (EDV)

EDV

The ejection fraction
= STROKE VOLUME
       EDV

emptying

filling
rate

filling
time

filling

mid-diastole

Ventricular filling takes place
during diastole. The volume
of blood entering = filling rate × filling time

end-systole
Ventricle at end of contraction
The amount of blood left
in the ventricle is the
end systolic volume (ESV)

ESV

Figure 1.3D Ventricular filling and cardiac output

13

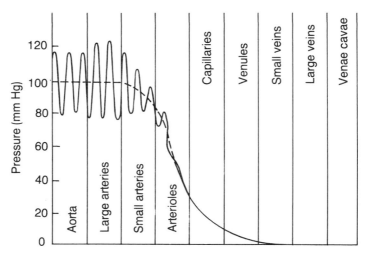

Figure 1.3E Pressures in different parts of the circulation

Lung perfusion

Lung perfusion is produced by the right ventricle working at relatively low pressure. The same equation applies as on the left:

$$RVO \times PVR = PAP$$

where PVR is pulmonary vascular resistance and PAP is pulmonary arterial pressure.

This is not often forced on our attention because the pulmonary arterial pressure cannot easily be measured.

The PAP becomes important when it is raised, as it is in chronic lung disease causing cor pulmonale or (rarely) in primary pulmonary hypertension. It is also raised in left ventricular failure. The back pressure from the failing left ventricle causes compensatory pulmonary arteriolar constriction and reduces lung perfusion, protecting the lungs from further increase in pressure and pulmonary oedema. This causes an increase in pulmonary arterial pressure, which can eventually cause the right ventricle to fail: congestive, or biventricular, heart failure (see Chapter 4.3).

HOMEOSTATIC MECHANISMS

We have added the two main homeostatic mechanisms in the model shown in Figure 1.3F:
(1)   the autonomic nervous system (Figure 1.3G);
(2)   the renin – angiotensin – aldosterone system (Figure 1.3H).

The autonomic nervous system

The behaviour of the cardiovascular system is regulated, to a great extent, by the competing, or balancing effects of the sympathetic and parasympathetic divisions of the autonomic nervous system.

Sympathetic tone

Sympathetic tone is increased by exercise; by a fall in systemic blood pressure (detected by baroreceptors in the carotid sinus and aortic arch) and by stress (the fight/flight mechanism).

The effects of increased sympathetic tone are complex. They can be divided into alpha- and beta-adrenergic effects, some of which are shown in Table 1.3A.

The alpha- and beta-effects can be further subdivided into $alpha_1$-, $alpha_2$-, $beta_1$- and $beta_2$-efects (see Figure 1.3I).

Table 1.3A Some alpha- and beta-adrenergic effects

	alpha-effects	*beta-effects*
	Vasoconstriction	Vasodilatation
	Intestinal muscle relaxation	Heart: increased force and rate; arrhythmias
	Pupillary dilatation	Bronchial relaxation
Noradrenaline	+ + +	+
Adrenaline	+	+ + +

Sympathetic activity causes increases in contractility (see below), heart rate and blood pressure (Figure 1.3J) and therefore in cardiac work. This results in an increase in the oxygen requirements of the myocardium. Another of its effects is to increase coronary perfusion by causing dilatation of the coronary arteries. It demands increased work at the same time as providing the wherewithal for it to be done.

15

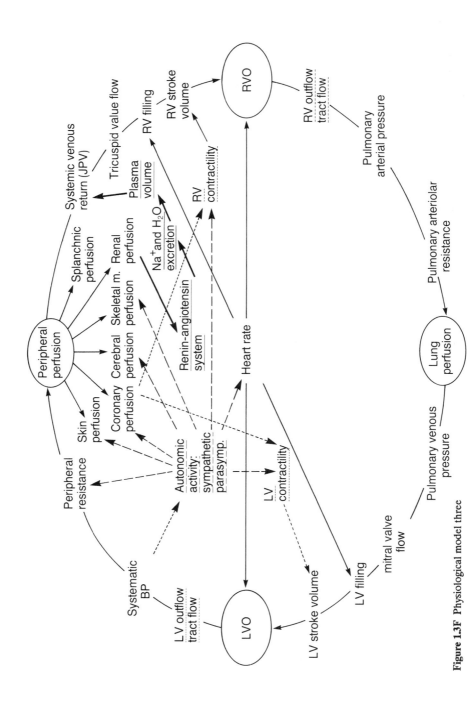

Figure 1.3F Physiological model three

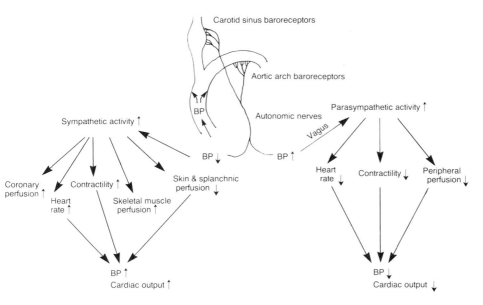

Figure 1.3G The autonomic nervous system

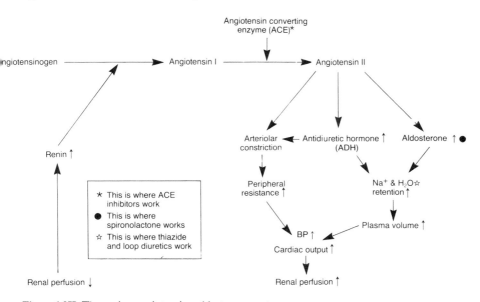

Figure 1.3H The renin – angiotensin – aldosterone system

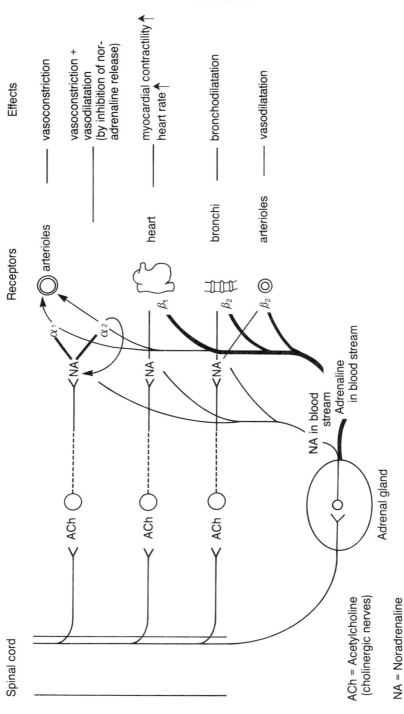

Figure 13I Alpha- and beta-effects of sympathetic nervous system

ACh = Acetylcholine (cholinergic nerves)

NA = Noradrenaline

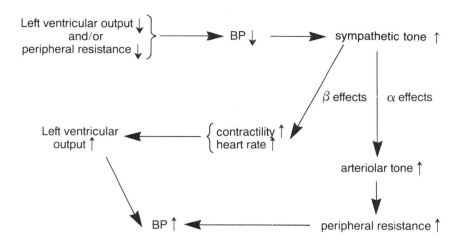

Figure 1.3J Sympathetic control of blood pressure

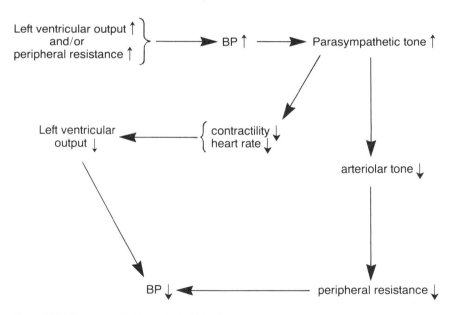

Figure 1.3K Parasympathetic control of blood pressure

Parasympathetic tone

Parasympathetic (vagal) tone is increased by rise in blood pressure (detected by baroreceptors in the carotid sinus and aortic arch); by depression/lethargy and by fear or pain (vaso-vagal attack). It causes bradycardia by slowing conduction at the S–A node and thus reduces cardiac output and blood pressure (Figure 1.3K).

Its effects are mediated by acetylcholine and are blocked by atropine. Atropine can correct a dangerous bradycardia by blocking the vagal effect and leaving the sympathetic effect unopposed. However, high vagal tone reduces cardiac work and discourages ventricular tachycardia, which are good reasons for using atropine with care.

Figure 1.3L shows the overall regulation of blood pressure.

The model shown in Figure 1.3F includes some other features of importance:

(1)   The left ventricular outflow tract:
   –   aortic valve;
   –   sub-valvar area.

(2)   The right ventricular outflow tract:
   –   pulmonary valve;
   –   sub-valvar (infundibular) area.

Ventricular contractility

This important concept is the pumping power of the heart and is the focus of attention in a number of disease processes and drug effects. It is responsible for the proportion of end diastolic volume ejected from the ventricle by each contraction: the ejection fraction.

Contractility depends on the health of the myocardium and on the availability of calcium ions within myocardial cells. An increase in contractility is called a positive inotropic effect. Increased ventricular filling, which stretches the myocardium, has a positive inotropic effect (the Frank–Starling mechanism) as also does sympathetic activity. Both these mechanisms come into play during exercise (Figure 1.3M).

Digoxin has a positive inotropic effect not mediated by the sympathetic system.

Contractility is decreased by decreased ventricular filling, by parasympathetic activity, by reduced coronary perfusion and by drugs, such as beta-blockers, which are therefore said to have a negative inotropic action.

All these effects are associated with the movement of calcium ions across the myocardial cell wall. An increase in available intracellular calcium ions increases the contractility of the myofibrils and also the oxygen requirement of the myocardium. The effects of calcium ions are shown in Figure 1.3N.

Contractility is reduced by any process which damages the myocardium, causing the myofibrils to be replaced by fibrous connective tissue. The most important such process occurs in ischaemic heart disease

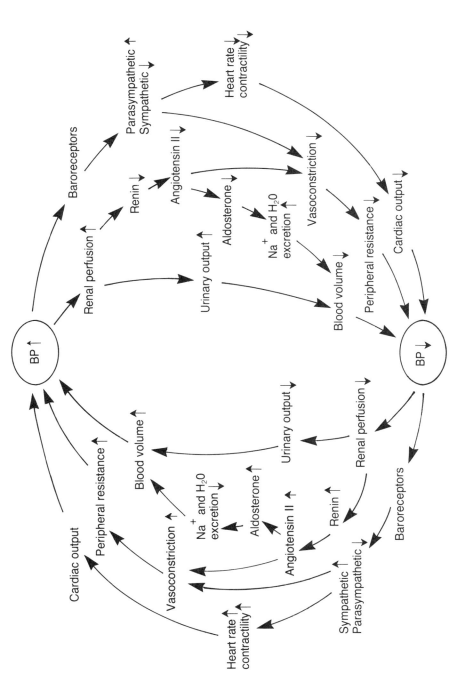

Figure 13L Overall regulation of blood pressure by autonomic nervous system and renin – angiotensin – aldosterone system

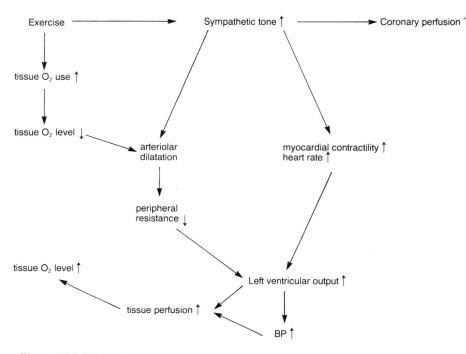

Figure 1.3M Effects of exercise

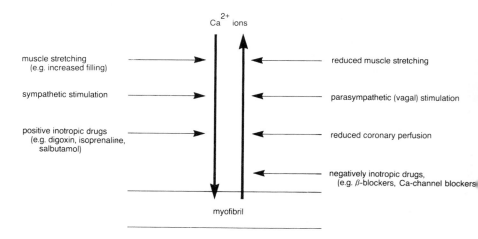

Figure 1.3N Ca^{2+}: effects and influences

Coronary artery perfusion

This takes place during diastole. It therefore depends on the diastolic blood pressure and on the length of diastole as well as on the patency of the coronary arteries.

Coronary perfusion is reduced by:
   low diastolic pressure
   rapid heart rate
   coronary atheroma.

Sympathetic activity causes:
   coronary artery dilatation
   increased diastolic pressure
   increased heart rate
   increased cardiac work.

The first two of these sympathetic effects increase coronary perfusion; the third reduces it. In health, the overall effect is an increase. If the coronary arteries are narrowed by atheroma, increased sympathetic activity may, on balance, reduce coronary perfusion, while increasing work.

Evidence for this is seen in the way stress and exercise cause angina and in the usefulness of beta-blockers in preventing it.

The workload of the heart

This depends on the volume of blood being moved and the pressure being exerted on it.

Overwork is more often a problem for the left ventricle than for the right because the pressures on the left are usually higher than on the right.

The work of the left ventricle (Figure 1.3O) can be seen in terms of output (stroke volume and heart rate) and blood pressure. The blood pressure is the product of cardiac output and the peripheral or systemic vascular resistance (SVR), sometimes called the afterload, to distinguish it from the other source of increased cardiac work: the venous return, or preload.

As we have already seen, the left ventricular output, working against the SVR produces the blood pressure:

$$LVO \times SVR = BP$$

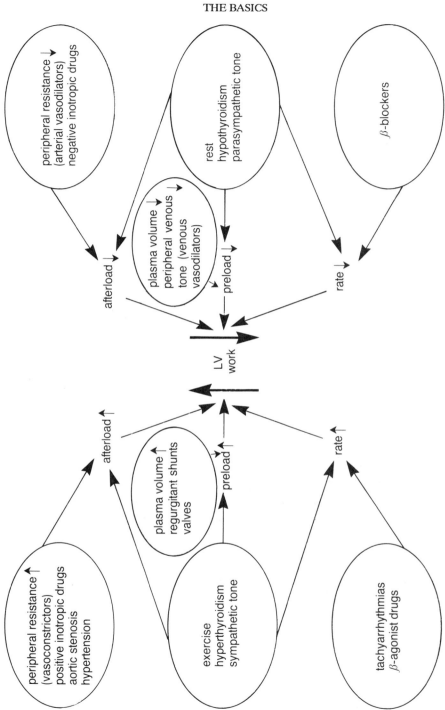

Figure 1.30 Left ventricular work

If the SVR increases, the left ventricle has to work harder to maintain a steady output and the blood pressure rises. This is what happens in exercise and also in hypertension.

Systolic pressure in the left ventricle is also increased by any increase in resistance in the outflow tract, such as occurs in aortic stenosis, which causes the heart to work harder to maintain its stroke volume.

Any prolonged increase in cardiac work results eventually in hypertrophy of the myocardium of the chamber affected.

Any increase in cardiac work requires an increase in coronary perfusion. If the capacity of the coronary arteries is limited by atheroma or spasm, then such an increase in perfusion may not be possible. This is why exercise and hypertension may precipitate angina in someone with ischaemic heart disease and why rest and beta-blockers relieve or prevent it. Many factors act in more than one way. For example a tachycardia demands increased work and causes decreased coronary perfusion; nitrates reduce preload (by veno-dilatation), afterload by reduction of SVR and also dilate the coronary arteries; sympathetic activity increases work but dilates the coronary arteries.

THE CONFLICT OF SURVIVAL MECHANISMS AND DISEASE PROCESSES

The basic homeostatic, or feedback mechanisms work well when applied to the needs of primitive man, in whom they originally developed, or in his modern counterpart, facing external threat.

Consider the two most likely emergencies:

Intense exertion

In intense exertion, which might be needed in hunting or in fighting or fleeing from an aggressor, dilatation of arterioles supplying active tissues and an immediate increase in sympathetic activity ensure:

(1) distribution of blood supply to where it is most needed (brain, heart, skeletal muscle);

(2) increase in cardiac output;

(3) reduction in fluid loss (resulting from reduced renal perfusion).

25

Haemorrhage

After haemorrhage, the sympathetic system continues to act, stimulated now by a fall in blood pressure. The reduction in cardiac output and renal perfusion triggers the renin – angiotensin system. This has a dual role:

(1) *immediately*, the vasopressor effect of angiotensin II helps to keep the blood pressure up in the short term;

(2) *later*, the increase in plasma volume allows the circulation to be maintained, while long-term reparative work takes place.

All this involves a massive increase in cardiac work and depends on a healthy myocardium as well as on structurally normal valves and vasculature.

Unfortunately, the body reacts as if every fall in blood pressure is due to haemorrhage. The same mechanisms are activated in acute myocardial infarction. By demanding an increase in work from the heart, when it is least able to cope with it, they are then distinctly unhelpful.

It is for this reason that a number of drugs have been developed to interfere with these mechanisms. More can be expected. At the time of writing, they include:

- beta-blockers, which interfere with the beta-effects of the sympathetic nervous system;
- anti-aldosterone agents;
- angiotensin-converting enzyme (ACE) inhibitors;
- calcium-channel blockers.

EFFECTS OF EXERCISE

This (Figure 1.3P) is the last of the physiological models. It is the same as that shown in Figure 1.3F but is designed to show how changes are propagated round the cardiovascular system, in this case, by exercise. Two main changes trigger the process:

(1) *first*, an increase in sympathetic activity;

(2) *later*, dilatation of skeletal muscle vessels in response to increasing levels of metabolites.

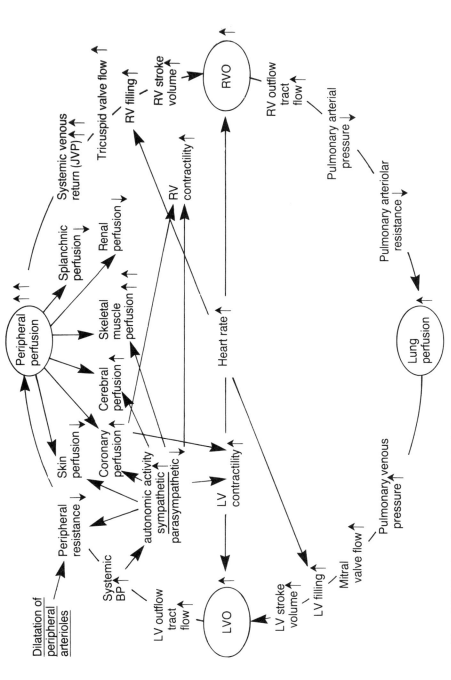

Figure 1.3P Exercise: effects on the physiological model

Increased sympathetic activity

Increased sympathetic activity causes:

(1)   increase in heart rate and contractility, both of which increase cardiac output: blood pressure rises;

(2)   dilatation of peripheral arterioles in coronary circulation, brain and skeletal muscle, increasing perfusion to these organs;

(3)   constriction of arterioles in the gut and kidneys, reducing their blood flow.

Dilatation of skeletal muscle vessels

This further increases muscle perfusion. The increase in perfusion and blood pressure and overall increase in cardiac output, cause a massive increase in left ventricular output and then of systemic venous return to the right ventricle. This is rapidly transmitted to the right side of the heart and the whole system becomes more dynamic with increased flow throughout.

HOW ARE THE PHYSIOLOGICAL MECHANISMS OBSERVED IN CLINICAL PRACTICE?

None of the physiological functions can be observed in isolation from the others: they all interrelate and depend on and affect each other. However, a knowledge of the contribution each makes to the clinical findings helps a great deal in interpreting symptoms, signs and investigation results.

Cardiac output is responsible for **perfusion**: peripheral; cerebral; renal; every organ and tissue. If it is normal, the individual has no (cardiac) limitations, physical or mental. If it is reduced, physical exertion is limited, mental confusion or loss of consciousness may occur, the skin may be cold, renal output reduced.

Contractility is intimately involved with cardiac output. Cardiac output cannot be normal without good contractility.

The **heart rate** is observed during clinical examination, when feeling the pulse and when listening to the heart. A history of rapid palpitations suggests a rapid heart rate. A history of dizzy spells or loss of consciousness could be evidence of a very fast or a very slow rate.

The **LV stroke volume** is estimated when feeling the pulse at the wrist or in the neck. It is also reflected in the pulse pressure: the difference between systolic and diastolic **blood pressure**. An excessively increased LV stroke volume may be observed visually and on palpation of the precordium. An abnormally small stroke volume is likely to be associated with a reduced cardiac output and some demonstrable pathology, such as an obstructive lesion like aortic stenosis or cardiomyopathy. These, in turn, give rise to symptoms, signs or ECG abnormalities (see later).

Normal **electrical activity** (Chapter 1.4) is demonstrated by a heart that is normal in rate and rhythm by the absence of a history suggesting arrhythmia and by a normal ECG.

Peripheral resistance and **blood pressure** are closely, though not invariably, linked (see above).

The **autonomic nervous system,** comprising both **sympathetic** and **parasympathetic** activity, is involved in regulating the pulse rate, skin colour and temperature (via **peripheral arteriolar tone**), sweating, pupil size and anxiety levels. If someone has a rapid pulse but is warm and pink, calm and relaxed, the tachycardia is probably not due solely to sympathetic activity.

The **right ventricular filling pressure** is that seen in the internal jugular vein. It is normally around zero and is therefore visible only when the patient lies flat.

The **left ventricular filling pressure** is deduced from the history and can be seen in the pulmonary veins on the chest X-ray. It is most unlikely to be raised if the patient is not breathless. A normal chest X-ray excludes raised pulmonary venous pressure at the time the film is taken but it may be intermittent and the radiological signs are often missed or misinterpreted.

Pulmonary perfusion can be deduced from a chest X-ray but cannot be demonstrated clinically.

The integrity of the **right** and **left outflow tracts** is revealed by the general behaviour of the rest of the cardiovascular system. If they are narrowed, flow through the system as a whole is reduced and there are signs of reduced output and perfusion as well as signs of the individual abnormalities themselves.

The heart sounds (Figure 1.3Q) are caused by the movement of the valves. The first sound is caused by the closure of the **mitral** and **tricuspid valves**. The mitral valve closes slightly before the tricuspid so that the sound is broad and not sharp.

The second sound is caused by the closure of the **aortic** and **pulmonary valves**. The aortic valve closes slightly before the pulmonary, so that the sound is split. This is a very narrow split and may be difficult to hear. It widens during inspiration, when the venous return to the right heart increases and the flow through the pulmonary valve, during systole, is prolonged. On expiration, the split disappears.

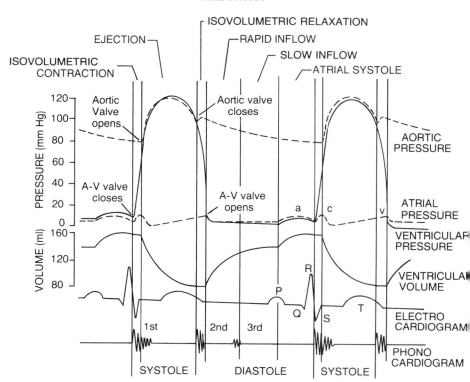

Figure 1.3Q Timing of events in the cardiac cycle

1.4
Electrophysiology

ELECTRICAL CONDUCTION IN MYOCARDIAL CELLS

There is an electrical potential (difference of charge) across the membrane of all cells. The function of the cells involves changes in the membrane potential. Some cells are able to generate electrochemical impulses at their membranes and transmit them as electrical signals. Myocardial cells are examples of cells which can do this.

When the cell is inactive, the membrane potential is said to be resting and the cell is polarised; that is, the outside of the cell is positively charged in relation to the inside (Figure 1.4A).

In myocardial cells, which are not acting as pacemakers, depolarisation is triggered by an electrical excitation wave. In pacemaker cells, depolarisation results from inherent rhythmicity: the natural rate of spontaneous discharge. The rate of the heart overall is controlled by the pacemaker with the fastest rate (normally, the S – A node).

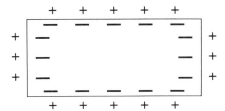

Figure 1.4A Cell charges at rest

In the normal heart, contraction follows rapid depolarisation, during which there is a sudden increase in permeability to sodium ions, which flood into the cell. The resulting change in charge across the membrane is called the action potential (Figure 1.4B). The membrane potential is now positive (depolarised).

Cardiac muscle is unique in that the positive action potential is maintained to form a plateau. This is made possible by the existence of slow calcium – sodium channels. This is an essential part of myocardial function because it is only during the action potential that the cell is refractory to further stimulation: an important safeguard against myocardial tetany.

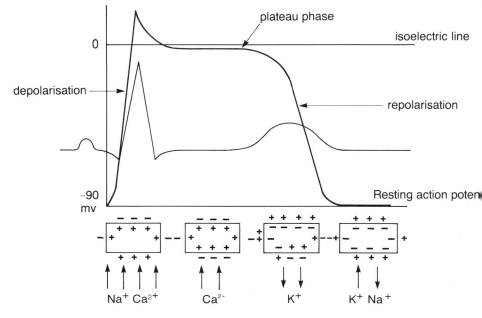

Figure 1.4B Diagram of action potential

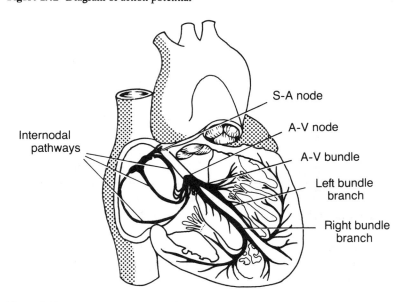

Figure 1.4C Conducting system of the heart

THE CONDUCTING SYSTEM OF THE HEART

Figure 1.4C is a diagram of the conducting system of the heart.

The normal cardiac cycle starts with an electrical impulse, or depolarisation wave, which arises in the sinus node, high up in the right atrium. This passes smoothly through the atria to the atrio-ventricular (A–V) node, causing depolarisation of the atria as it goes. This gives rise to the P wave on the ECG.

At the A–V node, there is a short delay which produces the P–R interval, before the impulse passes on into the ventricles via the bundle of His and the left and right bundle branches, which lie on either side of the ventricular septum.

The QRS complex is caused by the depolarisation of the ventricles. In the normal state, atrial depolarisation is always followed by ventricular depolarisation and therefore a QRS complex follows every P wave. Ventricular depolarisation always and only follows atrial depolarisation and therefore a P wave precedes every QRS complex.

The P wave reflects events in both atria. Normally, the right atrium begins to depolarise slightly before the left because the sinus node is in the right atrium (Figure 1.4D). The P waves from the two atria therefore overlap each other to produce a smooth, rounded deflection.

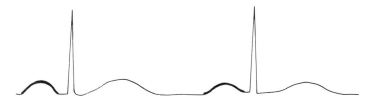

Figure 1.4D Normal P wave

If the right atrium is enlarged, as in cor pulmonale, depolarisation of the right atrium takes longer and the deflections from the two atria are more exactly superimposed to form a sharper, peaked deflection: the P pulmonale (Figure 1.4E).

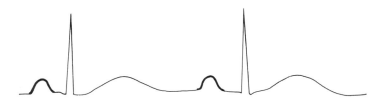

Figure 1.4E P pulmonale

If the left atrium is enlarged, as it is in mitral stenosis, depolarisation of the left atrium takes longer and the two elements of the P wave are spread to form the two-humped P mitrale (Figure 1.4F).

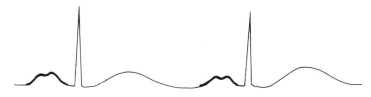

Figure 1.4F P mitrale

The length of the P – R interval depends on the degree of delay at the A – V node. It is normally between 0.1 and 0.2 sec (Figure 1.4G) or 2½ to five small squares. A longer delay than this is a sign of first degree heart block (Figure 1.4H).

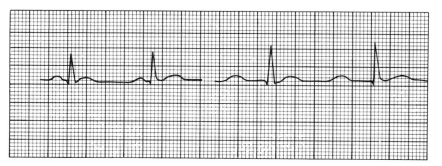

Figure 1.4G (left) Normal P – R interval
Figure 1.4H (right) Long P – R interval (first degree heart block)

An abnormally short P – R interval suggests that the depolarisation wave has bypassed the A – V node and taken a short cut through another part of the atrioventricular ring. This is what happens in the Wolff – Parkinson – White, or pre-excitation, syndrome (Figure 1.4I).

If the depolarisation wave cannot pass the A – V node, the ventricles contract at their own rate in response to a depolarisation wave originating either from the A – V node itself (junctional escape rhythm) or from a ventricular pacemaker (idioventricular rhythm). A junctional escape rhythm is characterised by narrow, normally shaped QRS complexes without regular preceding P waves and a rate of 50 – 60/min. An idioventricular rhythm results in broad QRS complexes not associated with P waves and a rate of 25/min.

The atria and ventricles are functioning independently of each other. This is third degree, or complete, heart block (Figure 1.4J).

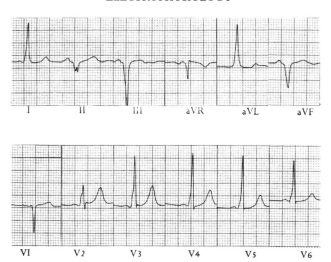

Figure 1.4I Wolff – Parkinson – White syndrome

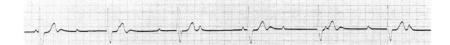

Figure 1.4J Third degree heart block

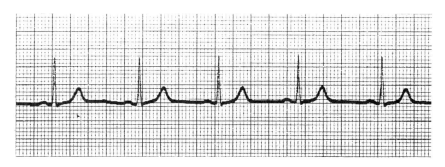

Figure 1.4K Normal QRS

The QRS complexes are caused by depolarisation of the ventricles. With normal conduction, they should not exceed 0.1 sec (Figure 1.4K).

If one of the His bundle branches fails to conduct, the depolarisation wave to that ventricle has to take a circuitous route via peripheral branches of the His – Purkinje network and is delayed. This causes a broadening of the QRS complex, which will be of a different shape depending on which bundle is affected (Figures 1.4L and 1.4M).

35

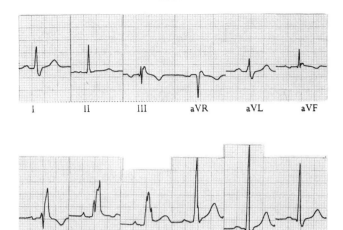

Figure 1.4L Right bundle branch block

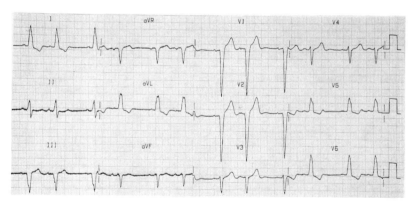

Figure 1.4M Left bundle branch block

Repolarisation of the ventricles results in the T wave, which follows every QRS complex.

The T wave is usually of the same general direction as the QRS complex which it follows. It is therefore normally upright in all the chest leads and in those limb leads where the QRS complex is positive.

PART 2:
CARDIAC DRUGS

2.1
Introduction

Drugs form the mainstay of treatment in cardiology. They are numerous, complex, highly effective and potentially dangerous. They contribute a great deal to the improved quality of life of patients with heart disease but also to the high level of iatrogenic morbidity.

None of us would want to practise without them and yet we are all made anxious by the knowledge that, unless used with extreme care, they can as easily make the patient worse as better. The phrase 'extreme care' seems, most of the time, to mean an unachievable level of knowledge and superhuman ability to predict the unpredictable. The aim of this section is to make the use of cardiac drugs a little less worrying for the doctor as well as safer and more effective for the patient. It contains two chapters:

Chapter 2.2: Hazards, Safety and Effectiveness;

Chapter 2.3: Sorting Out the Drugs.

2.2
Hazards, Safety and Effectiveness

HAZARDS

Cardiac drugs have great pharmacological power but apart from this there are other factors which render them particularly susceptible to potentially dangerous complications and side-effects. These include the following:

(1)   the conditions for which they are prescribed are chronic, often lifelong, and the drugs are therefore taken for very long periods, often many years;

(2)   many of the patients are elderly, or at least grow old during the course of treatment;

(3)   the drugs are often used in combination; it is not unusual for someone (quite properly) to be taking six or eight drugs at the same time (see Cameo);

(4)   it is sometimes difficult to distinguish symptoms and signs of disease from the effects of drug treatment;

(5)   the number of drugs, the way manufacturers produce them in combination in single preparations and the complexity of the pharmacology make it extremely difficult for the doctor to keep in mind all the facts relevant to prescribing.

CAMEO

Sam Bowen is 63. He has had moderate, benign, essential hypertension since his early forties and a grumbling duodenal ulcer for many years. He retired from his job as an HGV driver when he had his first myocardial infarct 5 years ago. Following that, he did part-time work as a storeman but had a further infarct 3 months ago. Since then he has had persistent angina. He has been taking atenolol and bendrofluazide since before his first infarct and takes ranitidine for his DU. He has been on warfarin since he was discharged from hospital 3 months ago. The angina is now reasonably well controlled on diltiazem, iso-sorbide mononitrate and a glyceryl trinitrate (GTN) spray.

His present medication is:
atenolol, 100 mg once a day
bendrofluazide, 2.5 mg once a day
ranitidine, 150 mg at night
diltiazem, 60 mg three times a day
isosorbide mononitrate, 20 mg three times a day
GTN sublingual spray as required
warfarin as per prothrombin time.

These factors have the following results:

- the condition for which the drug was originally prescribed may change over the course of time and the drug become inappropriate or ineffective;

- the necessary addition of other drugs may precipitate interactions, summations or side-effects;

- the patient may develop other diseases, for which other treatment is taken;

- increasing age of the patient may render the drug, or its dose, unsuitable;

- long-term prescribing is difficult to monitor and dosage regimes may become subtly altered in ways of which the doctor is unaware. (It is not uncommon to find that patients have forgotten why they are taking the drug, let alone the correct dose);

- unlike patients in hospital, those at home have supplies of drugs, often quite large. A patient may continue to take a drug which the doctor intended to stop, when prescribing another. Two similar or incompatible drugs are then being taken together;

- increasing age sometimes results in confusion, even with a well-established regimen;

- the doctor may be unaware of, or forget, the actions, side-effects or interactions of the drugs and the effects of overdosage. It is particularly difficult to remember what is in combined preparations; one of the constituents may be prescribed separately in addition or an incompatible drug be given inadvertently.

CAMEO

Harry Robson is 66. He was found to be mildly hypertensive when he was admitted to hospital with an acute myocardial infarction 18 months ago. He has taken atenolol, 100 mg daily since then. He has recently been in hospital for radiotherapy for a carcinoma of the bladder. Whilst in hospital he had several attacks of angina. The registrar sent him home with a prescription for nifedipine SR, 20 mg twice a day and GTN sublingual tablets, 500 mcg to be taken as required. His wife called the doctor when he had a fall. His blood pressure was 104/62, standing. The drug dosage was reduced and he felt much better. His blood pressure rose to 125/80.

He is now taking:

atenolol, 50 mg daily
nifedipine, 5 mg three times a day
GTN sublingual tablets, 300 mcg as required.

HOW MAY THE DOCTOR ACHIEVE PEACE OF MIND WHEN PRESCRIBING CARDIAC DRUGS?

(1)   Have a clear understanding of the main groups of drugs and allocate every one to its group (see later).

This is made difficult by the pharmaceutical companies, who dislike doctors labelling the new wonder drug as 'just another beta-blocker'. However, it is essential for safe practice and reduces the total number of facts which have to be remembered, since many of the actions and interactions of drugs apply to all members of a group.

(2)   Revise the physiology of the cardiovascular system and maintain a picture of the way in which drugs affect it. This enables the doctor safely to rely on commonsense rather than having to memorise a huge number of rules.

(3)   Devise a simple code of practice, or prescribing protocol, if possible shared by others working in the practice.

The version given below is one possible form of such a code of practice. Ideally, every doctor, or group working together, should devise their own to suit their own particular needs.

CODE FOR PRESCRIBING CARDIAC DRUGS

General

(1)   The specific indication for each drug is noted in the patient's records (e.g.'nifedipine for angina').

(2)   A note is made of particular side-effects or interactions to be watched for in that patient (e.g. 'watch for hypotension: normal BP & already taking nitrate').

(3)   Only one drug from a group to be prescribed (e.g. not nifedipine *and* diltiazem) (see Figure 2.2A).

(4)   No combination drugs will be used without good reason and a note made in the patient's records of the constituents.

(5)   An indication is made in the records as to whether a newly prescribed drug is to be taken as well as or instead of those previously prescribed (e.g.'add nifedipine').

(6)   Dosage is deliberately reviewed at intervals to take account of response and side-effects as well as the effects of increasing age and intercurrent disease. The review is noted in the records.

(7)   A note is kept of any regular tests required (e.g. 'BP every 6 months'; 'U & Es once a year').

(8)   A summary of drugs is noted in a list at frequent intervals and rewritten in full every time a change is made.

(9)   Every patient is asked, at all times, to carry a card with a list of all the drugs he is taking, with their dosage. Everything he is taking must be on the list. The dose is written in English and instructions are carefully worded, avoiding phrases such as 'as directed', 'as before', 'when needed'.

(10)   The card is checked and updated every time the patient is seen.

(11)   The patient knows what each drug is for and how it should be taken (e.g. 'use spray as soon as chest pain starts').

Specific

Draw up a drug treatment protocol to be used for all common conditions. It helps if it is as detailed as possible and includes names of specific drugs, dosages and warnings. It can form part of an overall practice management protocol for the condition.

Such a code must be flexible enough to allow variation in particular patients as long as any departure from it is recorded in the patient's notes. It in no way restricts any doctor, unless he chooses that it should, as he is free to prescribe outside it if he wishes to do so. It has some important advantages. It makes prescribing decisions quicker, easier, safer and more consistent; it makes it possible for everyone in the practice to know what is, or should be, happening to every patient; it can form a baseline, a default procedure, which is especially valuable when a patient's usual doctor is not available; it enables doctors to become familiar with individual drugs; it can be easily modified in the light of advances in treatment, opinion or experience; it allows all the partners to benefit from the particular expertise or interest of each and to share new information gleaned from reading or

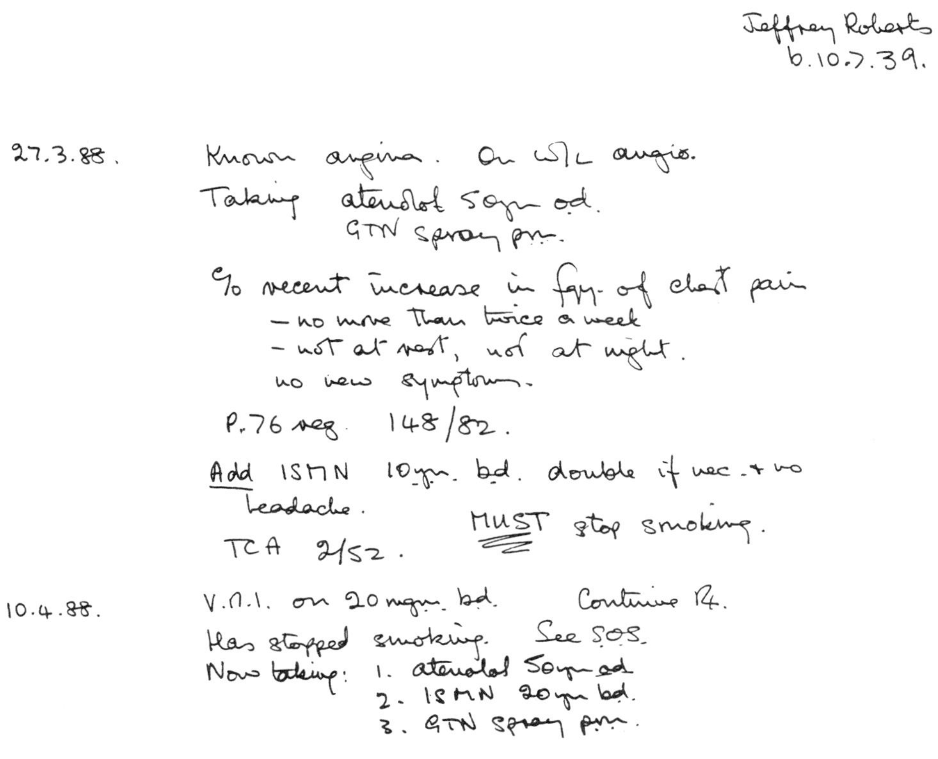

Jeffrey Roberts
b.10.7.39.

27.3.88. Known angina. On W/L angio.
Taking atenolol 50ym od.
GTN spray prn.

% recent increase in fqy. of chest pain
— no more than twice a week
— not at rest, not at night.
no new symptoms.

P.76 reg. 148/82.

Add ISMN 10ym. bd. double if nec. + no
headache.
TCA 2/52. MUST stop smoking.

10.4.88. V.N.I. on 20mgm bd. Continue Rx.
Has stopped smoking. See SOS.
Now taking: 1. atenolol 50ym od
2. ISMN 20ym bd.
3. GTN spray prn.

Figure 2.2A Example of hand-written notes

EXAMPLE OF PRESCRIBING PROTOCOL

Angina: two weeks between each addition.

(1)   Sublingual nitrate: aerosol spray: as required.
      (*Risk* of headache and postural hypotension.)

(2)   Oral nitrate: isosorbide mononitrate: 10 mg three times a day
      increasing gradually to 80 mg three times a day if needed. Last dose
      before 8 p.m.
      (*Risk* of headache and postural hypotension.)

(3)   Beta-blocker: atenolol 50 mg once a day, increasing to 100 mg if
      needed.
      (*Not* if history of asthma; *care* if risk of heart failure.)

(4)   Calcium-channel blocker: diltiazem 60 mg twice a day, increasing to
      120 mg three times a day if needed.
      (*Watch* for hypotension and increasing fatigue due to low output as
      drugs are added.)

---

attending meetings or courses and it ensures, as far as possible, that patients receive and take, in the optimum way, the drugs which are most likely to benefit them, with a minimum of side-effects and risk.

A code of practice cannot include all aspects of medication and there are many problems which it cannot easily cover. It is difficult to monitor what the patient is taking, especially if he is also attending one or more hospital out-patient clinics, or is getting old and muddled.

WHAT QUESTIONS ARISE?

(1)   Does the GP know when a patient is given a new drug in hospital outpatients?

(2)   Does the hospital doctor know what the patient is already taking?

(3)   Does each hospital doctor know what is being prescribed in other clinics, either in the same hospital or somewhere else? (No-one ever knows what is being prescribed to whom in the STD clinics!)

(4)   Does the patient know: what the drug is for; how to take it: when, as well as by what route; what side-effects to expect/ watch for/ report: at once/ as soon as possible/ at next visit; whether a drug is to be taken as well as or instead of other drugs and if it is to be taken for a

particular symptom, how often should it be repeated; how soon will it take effect; is there a maximum dose; who should he tell if it does not help?

(5)   Is the patient also taking over-the-counter medicines?

WHAT SHOULD BE DONE TO ENSURE SAFE PRESCRIBING?

All instructions should be first spoken and then written down for the patient to take home. This has nothing to do with intelligence or grasp of what he has been told. The most intelligent people simply forget information, especially if too much is given at once or they are anxious or distracted. Patient advice leaflets can be used (see Figure 2.2B).

Side-effects must be sought deliberately. Many people do not think to tell the doctor about lack of energy, nightmares, constipation, breathlessness on exertion, cold extremities or impotence unless specifically asked. Headache and depression are common symptoms and also common side-effects. Some side-effects may be unavoidable and worth putting up with but it is important that they are recognised for what they are so that the patient can share in the decision to continue with the drug and come to terms with its effects. Some symptoms may be unrelated to the drugs. These too have to be sorted out.

```
Name of patient..John Smith..................
Name of drug....Frusemide.....................
Size of tablet..40 mgm......................
Daily dose...120 mgm.....(3 tablets).........
When to take it...2 in the morning...........
            ...1 at midday..................
How long for...indefinitely..................
What it is for..1. to reduce congestion breathlessness
            .2. to make you pass more urine.
Likely side effects..None.....................
See doctor if..breathlessness increases.......
Next appointment...March....................
Special remarks:

        Take care not to run out.
        Ask for a repeat prescription
            in good time.
```

Figure 2.2B Patient advice leaflet

2.3
Sorting Out the Drugs

INTRODUCTION

In this chapter, we describe the groups of drugs commonly used in the treatment of heart disease, giving examples of individual drugs, but we assume that each doctor will decide for himself which to have in his own personal formulary.

List of groups of drugs described

Cardiac glycosides	digoxin
Diuretics:	thiazides
	loop diuretics
	potassium-sparing diuretics
Beta-blockers	
Vasodilators:	nitrates
	calcium-channel blocking agents
	ACE inhibitors
	adrenergic neurone-blocking drugs
	alpha-adrenoceptor-blocking drugs
	direct-acting vasodilators
Anti-arrhythmics	
Anti-clotting agents	

Information

Each group of drugs is treated similarly. First it is defined and then its effects are described. The drug(s) are described in answer to a series of questions such as:

How does it work?
Who should take it/not take it?
What dose?
Side-effects – what precautions should you take?
Toxicity – what may happen and what can you do?
What preparations are available?
Which to choose?

At the end of each group any special points that it is important always to bear in mind are set out in a box.

DIGOXIN

What is it?

It is a synthetic cardiac glycoside, chemically related to oestrogens and other steroids such as spironolactone.

What does it do?

It is a positive inotropic agent. This means that it increases the force of contraction (contractility) of heart muscle. It also has a vagal effect in slowing the heart. Its main effects are:
-   to slow conduction at the A – V node;
-   to increase cardiac output by increasing contractility.

The effect on conduction means that, as long as the rhythm is atrial, i.e. the impulses leading to ventricular depolarisation arise in the atria and pass through the A – V node, digoxin slows the heart rate. It may not slow the atrial rate. In fact, it may increase it, making atrial fibrillation more likely to develop in someone with atrial flutter or who is in sinus rhythm but who has a tendency to paroxysmal fibrillation. It has no useful effect on patients with ventricular rhythms and may be dangerous.

The effect on contractility means that it may increase cardiac output in patients with heart failure.

Digoxin causes ECG changes (Figure 2.3A): S – T segment depression or 'sagging' and flat T waves, even at therapeutic blood levels. At toxic levels, any arrhythmia can occur.

How does it work?

In terms of myocardial physiology, digoxin is something of a paradox, having apparently contradictory effects on different aspects of cardiac function. Its effect on SA node firing and on A – V conduction result from increased vagal tone. Its effect on contractility results from an increase in the movement of calcium ions across the myocardial cell membrane into the cell due to inhibition of the sodium pump.

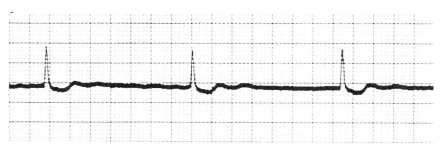

Figure 2.3A ECG changes caused by digoxin treatment

Who should take it?

Atrial fibrillation is the main indication. It is sometimes used for other arrhythmias, e.g. supraventricular tachycardia (SVT). It is not often used in the treatment of heart failure in the UK unless atrial fibrillation is also present.

Who should not take it?

Anyone with the following conditions should avoid digoxin, unless closely supervised by a cardiologist:

–   Wolff – Parkinson – White syndrome
–   Hypertrophic obstructive cardiomyopathy (HOCM)
–   Risk of digoxin overdose
–   Certain complex arrhythmias
–   Heart block
–   Left ventricular hypertrophy (LVH) due to hypertension
–   Other drugs inhibiting A – V conduction (e.g. verapamil, beta-blockers, amiodarone)

Care is needed in situations where there is increased likelihood of toxicity: renal failure, hypokalaemia; where there is increased sensitivity to the drug: great age or frailty, hypokalaemia, hypothyroidism, chronic pulmonary disease; where the myocardium is likely to be irritable: recent myocardial infarction, atrial fibrillation associated with hyperthyroidism, myocarditis; where increased contractility, requiring increased oxygen supply, is undesirable: ischaemic heart disease, severe ventricular hypertrophy, valvular stenosis and where delayed A – V conduction is undesirable: sinus brady-cardia, A – V conduction defects. From this list it can be seen that many of the potential risks of digoxin can be avoided by checking the blood urea and electrolytes before prescribing. A good maxim is:

DIGOXIN SHOULD NEVER BE PRESCRIBED UNLESS THE
BLOOD UREA IS KNOWN

What dose?

There is no indication for rapid digitalisation in general practice.

Gradual digitalisation: 125 – 250 mcg twice daily for 5 – 7 days.

Maintenance dose: 62.5 – 250 mcg daily is usual but the dose must be monitored to avoid toxicity. A useful rule is to aim to keep the resting pulse rate down to less than 90 but above 60 per min.

Less is needed if the blood urea is raised; if the serum potassium is low; in the lean and in the aged.

The plasma digoxin level can be a guide to dosage but the optimum level varies between individuals. Blood should be taken 8 hours after the last dose.

Digoxin is excreted unchanged by the kidneys. The serum half-life of digoxin is 36 hours and it is not usually necessary to take it more often than once a day. However, in some people, an undesirable dip occurs towards the end of each 24 hours and a twice daily dose may then be more appropriate.

Digitoxin is broken down by the liver and may therefore be a better choice for a patient with renal failure. The serum half-life of digitoxin is 6 – 7 days, which makes toxicity much more difficult to manage. It should not be taken more often than once a day.

Digoxin and digitoxin are cumulative and a very slight overdose carries over from one day to the next, eventually culminating in insidious toxicity which may be undetected but potentially very dangerous. A traditional way to minimise this risk is to omit the drug altogether on one day a week. This remains a useful safeguard in those in whom continuing level of dose is not crucial.

Toxicity

What may happen?

Toxic effects may occur with a very small dose in a sensitive individual and can be life-threatening. The most important factor is for the doctor to maintain a high index of suspicion of the possibility. It is easy to miss for several reasons:

- the patient may have been taking the drug in the same dose for many years;

- toxicity may develop gradually over many weeks and be attributed to a general deterioration in health;

- if it develops suddenly in association with another unconnected problem, such as a feverish illness causing dehydration and a raised blood urea, the symptoms are likely to be blamed entirely on the acute condition;

- some of the signs, e.g. the tachyarrhythmia, may mimic the condition for which the drug was originally given and there is a danger that the dose may be increased in the presence of toxicity.

Digoxin toxicity may be precipitated in a patient on a well established maintenance dose by a number of factors:

(1)   the addition to the regime of another drug, such as a diuretic, which lowers the serum potassium or raises the blood urea;

(2)   renal failure due to any cause;

(3)   intercurrent illness causing dehydration and/or raised blood urea. Raised blood urea leads to digoxin toxicity which causes vomiting with consequent dehydration – this is a vicious circle.

Signs of toxicity include anorexia, nausea, vomiting, loss of weight, bradycardia and tachyarrhythmias.

CAMEO

Violet Bonnet is 74. She first developed atrial fibrillation many years ago and has been well controlled on digoxin 125 mcg daily.

She is usually a sprightly lady and lives on her own. She started to lose her appetite about 6 weeks ago and has felt nauseated in the mornings. She has obviously lost weight. She began to vomit occasionally and her doctor referred her to the medical oupatient clinic for investigation, thinking that she might have intra-abdominal malignant disease. She became dehydrated and had a raised blood urea. Whilst she was waiting for her appointment, she ran out of digoxin tablets. Within a few days, the nausea and vomiting subsided and gradually her appetite returned.

What to do?

Stop the drug.
Give fluids.
Take blood for urea and electrolytes.
Admit to hospital if severely affected.

What preparations are available?

Digoxin tablets: 62.5mcg; 125 mcg; 250 mcg.
Digitoxin tablets: 100 mcg.

What are the interactions with other drugs?

Increased toxicity may be caused by any drug which reduces potassium: e.g. carbenoxolone or diuretics.
Reduced absorption may be caused by cholestyramine and colestipol.

POINTS

In digoxin therapy:

 – watch out for toxicity
   – in the elderly
   – in dehydration

 – check urea and electrolytes if unwell

 – beware of anorexia, nausea, weight loss

DIURETICS

What are they?

They are a group of drugs which increase urinary output.

What do they do?

(1)   All reduce circulating blood volume, by increasing renal excretion of water and sodium ions. This has the effect of reducing venous return to the heart and therefore of right ventricular output and pulmonary blood flow. This relieves pulmonary oedema but it is not an immediate effect. It will also reduce peripheral oedema, which has developed as a result of congestive heart failure.

(2)   The loop diuretics, like frusemide, have an immediate venodilatory effect (Figure 2.3B). This causes pooling of blood in the peripheral, systemic veins and very quickly reduces venous return to the right heart, blood flow to the lungs and pulmonary oedema.

(3)   Thiazide diuretics, in small doses, reduce blood pressure in hypertension by increasing sodium excretion.

(4)   Thiazides and loop diuretics both have a stimulating effect on the renin–angiotensin system, triggered by the fall in serum sodium levels and by the reduction in circulating blood volume which they cause (see Figure 2.3C).

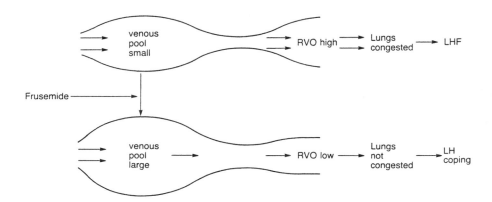

Figure 2.3B Venodilatory effects of frusemide

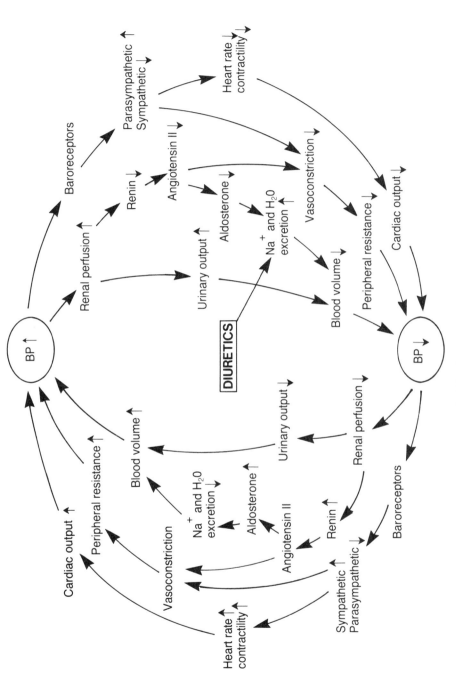

Figure 2.3C Effects of diuretics on the physiological control of blood pressure

How do they work?

Thiazides act on the distal tubules (Figure 2.3D), preventing resorption of water and sodium and potassium ions. They may also have a mild vasodilator effect.

Loop diuretics (e.g. frusemide) act on Henle's loop (Figure 2.3D) and also prevent reabsorption of water and of sodium and potassium ions. They are more powerful diuretics than the thiazides. Frusemide has a powerful and rapid venodilatory effect.

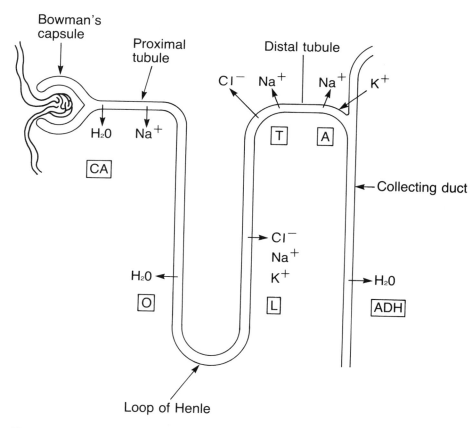

Figure 2.3D Nephron showing the site of action of diuretics
Key: CA = carbonic anhydrase inhibitors (e.g. diamox)
O = osmotic diuretics (e.g. mannitol)
L = loop diuretics (e.g. frusemide)
T = thiazides
A = potassium-sparing diuretics (aldosterone antagonists)
ADH = antidiuretic hormone

Potassium-sparing diuretics: amiloride, triamterene, spironolactone. These have only a weak diuretic effect. They are used in combination with thiazides or loop diuretics to try to avoid potassium depletion.

ACE inhibitors also act as mild, potassium-retaining diuretics by a mechanism similar to the action of spironolactone: by interrupting the renin – angiotensin – aldosterone system.

Who should take them?

All the diuretics are used with great effect in congestive heart failure and in pure left heart failure. Their use in pure right-sided heart failure is less straightforward (see p.209).

Thiazides are used in the treatment of mild hypertension but their position is not secure and they must be used in small doses if they are not to do more harm than good.

Who should not take them?

DIURETICS SHOULD NOT BE USED FOR THE TREATMENT OF PERIPHERAL OEDEMA WHICH IS NOT DUE TO HEART FAILURE.

Dependent oedema, due to stasis, is common and affects people who are otherwise well. Diuretics may initially have an apparently beneficial effect in reducing it but it rebounds if treatment is stopped. This makes it difficult to persuade patients to limit themselves to a small dose, taken intermittently, which might be safer. It also makes it likely that the drug will be taken for extremely long periods, maybe years.

It is the long-term administration of diuretics which is dangerous. They have an adverse effect on lipids and theoretically increase the risk of ischaemic heart disease; they cause hyperuricaemia and may precipitate gout; they aggravate glucose intolerance and may precipitate diabetes; they cause potassium depletion, with serious consequences in some people and they affect the renin – angiotensin – aldosterone system in a complex manner with the paradoxical result of increasing fluid retention and cardiac work.

Diuretics must be used with caution in people with renal failure. Frusemide may cause fewer problems than the thiazides. Thiazides and loop diuretics may reduce the serum potassium and thereby render the patient more susceptible to digoxin toxicity.

Which to choose?

Hypertension: (see p.234)

Thiazides in small doses
e.g.   2.5 mg bendrofluazide
        12.5 mg hydrochlorothiazide.

Mild to moderate heart failure: (see p.216)

Thiazide in combination with a potassium-sparing diuretic such as Dyazide:
        hydrochlorothiazide 25 mg ⎱
        triamterene 50 mg   ⎰

Severe or resistant heart failure: (see p.216)

Frusemide 40mg daily and upwards.

   If a small dose is all that is required, then it can be given in a single morning dose in combination with a potassium-sparing diuretic such as Frumil (frusemide 40 mg with amiloride 5 mg).
   If larger doses are required, then the frusemide has to be given separately and in divided doses:
e.g.   frusemide   80 mg in the morning
                     40 mg at mid-day;
        amiloride   10 mg in the morning.

   This avoids the problem of increasing both drugs by the same amount and also provides some protection against fluid overload during the night.

Acute left ventricular failure:

Frusemide 20–40 mg i.v. **SLOWLY** or 40 mg by mouth, followed by overall review (see p.216).

Side-effects

–   Hypokalaemia is not usually a problem when small doses are used, as in hypertension. It is avoided in other patients by using thiazides and loop diuretics in combination with potassium-sparing diuretics. Potassium supplements are not required unless a very large dose is being used. Patients should be encouraged to eat foods high in potassium, e.g.

bananas and other fruits and juices.

The symptoms and signs of hypokalaemia include muscular weakness, arrhythmias, digoxin toxicity and cardiac arrest.

– Postural hypotension may be a problem especially in the elderly.

– Gout: an attack may be precipitated in a susceptible individual.

– Diabetes: may be more difficult to control or precipitated in anyone with impaired glucose tolerance.

– Impotence.

– Lethargy.

CAMEO

At 78, Mary Pont is obese and immobile and has many complaints which are difficult to disentangle. They include breathlessness, difficulty in walking, rheumatic pains and constipation. She has been admitted to hospital a number of times and is generally considered to have had a small myocardial infarct on one occasion and perhaps a small CVA on another. She takes chlorthiazide because it was thought her breathlessness might be due to heart failure, some prescribed and some over-the-counter analgesics and a small dose of a benzodiazipine as a hypnotic.

After a particularly bad spell of cold weather, she became worse in all respects and was unable to get out of bed because of general weakness and unsteadiness. She said she had not had her bowels open for three weeks and had not eaten for two days. The community nurse asked the doctor to call when Mrs Pont started vomiting. She looked no different from her usual rather miserable self but her abdomen was distended and she was dehydrated. She was admitted to hospital where her serum potassium was found to be 2.1 mmol/l.

What precautions should you take?

Always use the smallest effective dose, especially in the elderly.

Check blood urea and electrolytes before starting and regularly during treatment, more frequently if high doses are being used or renal function is suspect.

POINTS

Use diuretics sparingly:

- use the mildest appropriate drug and smallest effective dose

- do not use for trivial reasons

- consider reducing or stopping where possible

- watch out for electrolyte imbalance

BETA-BLOCKERS

What are they?

A group of drugs which block the beta-adrenergic receptors of the sympathetic nervous system. These are mediated by adrenaline and are of most importance in the heart, bronchi and peripheral blood vessels.

The beta-receptors can be divided into $beta_1$-receptors, which are found in the heart, and $beta_2$-receptors, which are found in the bronchial and vascular smooth muscle.

How do they work?

Non-selective beta-blockers block both $beta_1$ and $beta_2$ receptors.
Cardioselective beta-blockers, at low doses, are relatively $beta_1$-specific.

Some also have an partial agonist activity (PAA). These simultaneously block and stimulate the receptors. If there is enhanced sympathetic tone the blockade dominates. (For the effects of this, see later.)

At a cellular level, beta-blockers reduce the concentration of intracellular calcium ions, altering the pattern of their movement across the cell membranes (see p.20)

What do they do?

The effects can be considered under the following headings.

Reduced myocardial contractility

Reduced stroke volume and cardiac output.
Exacerbation of pre-existing heart failure.
Reduced peripheral perfusion and exacerbation of symptoms of peripheral vascular disease.

Reduced heart rate

Reduced cardiac output.
Increased coronary perfusion by prolonging diastole.
Aggravation of heart block.

The combined effect of reduced contractility and reduced heart rate in reducing cardiac workload, is to reduce myocardial oxygen requirements. This explains the effectiveness of beta-blockers in the treatment of angina.

Smooth muscle spasm

(1)   Bronchospasm.
(2)   Peripheral vasoconstriction:
    −   increased peripheral resistance;
    −   reduced peripheral perfusion;
    −   exacerbation of symptoms of pre-existing peripheral vascular disease.

Increased refractory period of myocardial cells

This is especially important in the A−V node. The reduced excitability results in reduced incidence of some arrhythmias.

Reduced renin levels

Reduced blood pressure

This response is by mechanisms which are at present obscure.

Who should take them?

Patients with:

Angina: treatment of choice in patients with no contra-indications (see p.169)

Hypertension: first choice for most patients (but see p.234).

Arrhythmias: still have a place in the treatment of SVT but have been replaced by other drugs for most arrhythmias (see p.250).

Need for secondary prevention following acute myocardial infarction:
Propranolol, timolol and metoprolol have been shown to reduce morbidity and mortality after infarction for at least 2 years by reducing the incidence of sudden death and of reinfarction.

Who should not take them?

Anyone with: asthma
                    heart failure
                    insulin dependent diabetes
                    peripheral vascular disease

bradyarrhythmias, such as heart block
acute myocardial infarction
hypertriglyceridaemia.

In all these conditions there are exceptions: situations where beta-blockers may be beneficial, if carefully monitored. For instance, they are increasingly being used in the management of acute myocardial infarction, when the patient is being monitored in hospital.

Side-effects

- Central effects: fatigue, sleep disturbance, nightmares, depression, impotence.

- Reduced cardiac output: heart failure, reduced exercise tolerance, reduced peripheral perfusion, hypotension.

- Smooth muscle spasm:
  - bronchospasm
  - peripheral vasoconstriction: cold extremities, chilblains, intermittent claudication, rest pain, gangrene.

If side-effects are troublesome but not serious, it is worth trying a beta-blocker of a different type before abandoning this group of drugs.

CAMEO

Harry Warner is 62. He came to the surgery on Friday afternoon for a routine check of his hypertension. He started taking propranolol 40 mg three times a day 2 weeks ago. He said he was well but had recently become short of breath on exercise and at night. There were no abnormal physical signs. His blood pressure was 158/94. It was too late to have a chest X-ray and so, thinking he might be developing left ventricular failure, the doctor added frusemide 40 mg to his regime. Over the weekend, he became acutely breathless and the emergency doctor was called. He was distressed and had scattered rhonchi throughout both lung fields. The bronchospasm was relieved by inhaled salbutamol. He gave no history of asthma but had had attacks of winter 'bronchitis' from time to time. The breathlessness resolved when the beta-blocker was stopped.

Which to choose?

This is a large group of drugs, with more similarities than differences. It is useful to become familiar with a few, representing one from each main group, and stick with them.

Cardioselective

> Acebutolol
> Atenolol
> Metoprolol.

(1)   None are completely beta$_1$-specific, especially at higher doses, and the risk of bronchospasm is still present.

(2)   They have little advantage in patients with problems with peripheral perfusion as reduction in cardiac output is more important than peripheral vasoconstriction.

Water-soluble

> Atenolol
> Nadolol
> Sotalol.

These are less likely to enter the brain and cause central depressant effects, sleep disturbance and nightmares.

Partial agonist activity (PAA)

> Acebutolol
> Oxprenolol
> Pindolol.

These are less likely to cause bradycardia and cold extremities but the dose may be difficult to determine. The sympathomimetic effect is directly related to dose and increases throughout the dose range (see Figure 2.3E). The beta-blockade reaches a peak and no further increase in effect follows further increase in dose. Therefore, above a critical dose, which may be different for every patient, the sympathomimetic effect may outweigh the beta-blockade and produce an effect opposite to the one desired. This group may be best avoided, especially in the treatment of hypertension, unless a fixed low dose is used.

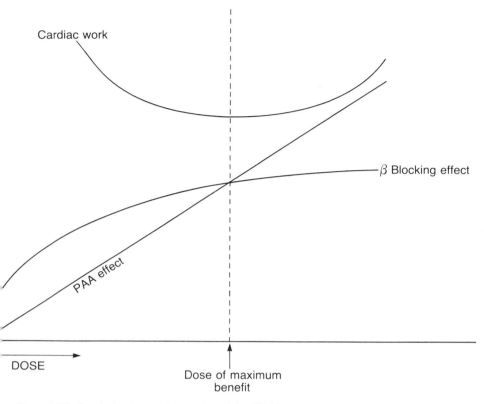

Figure 2.3E Graph showing partial agonist activity (PAA)

Short-acting (also available as slow-release preparations)

  Metoprolol
  Oxprenolol
  Propranolol.

These are metabolised by the liver.

Long-acting

  Acebutolol
  Nadolol.

These are excreted by the kidneys.

63

Interactions with other drugs

The most important one is verapamil. Both drugs are cardiac depressants and the combination may cause asystole.

Insulin-dependent diabetics rely on the action of adrenaline to provide them with the warning symptoms of hypoglycaemia. These may be masked by beta-blockers.

POINTS

With beta-blockers:

- beware a history of asthma or 'bronchitis'

- watch for heart failure

- peripheral vascular disease may be made worse

	PAA	MSA	Elimination	Plasma half-life (hours)	Oral dose	Tablet size (mg)	Slow release preparation
Cardioselective							
Atenolol (Tenormin)	–	–	R	6 – 9	50 – 100 mg once daily	50, 100	N/A
Metoprolol (Betaloc)	–	+	H	3 – 4	50 – 100 mg three times a day	50, 100	Betaloc SA 200 mg once daily
Acebutolol (Sectral)	+	+	R + H	6	100 – 200 mg three times a day Max 1200 mg daily	100, 200, 400	–
Non-cardioselective							
Propranolol (Inderal)	–	+	H	2 – 6	40 – 80 mg three times a day Max 320 mg daily	10, 40, 80, 160	Half-Inderal LA 80 mg once daily. Inderal LA 160 mg once daily
Oxprenolol (Trasicor)	+	+	H	2	20 – 80 mg three times a day Max 480 mg daily	20, 40, 80	Slow Trasicor 160 mg once daily
Sotalol (Beta-Cardone)	–	–	R	15 – 17	80 – 160 mg once or twice daily. Max 600 mg daily	40, 80, 160, 200	N/A
Timolol (Blocadren)	+/–	–	H	4 – 6	10 mg three times a day. Max 60 mg daily	10	–

PAA = Partial agonist activity
MSA = Membrane stabilising activity: anti-arrhythmic
R = Renal excretion: water-soluble drugs eliminated by kidneys. Care needed in renal failure
H = Hepatic breakdown: fat-soluble drugs broken down by liver. Have short half-life

VASODILATORS

What are they?

This is a large group of drugs with widely differing pharmacological properties. It includes a number of chemically unrelated compounds, which have different modes of action but which have in common the ability to cause dilatation of peripheral blood vessels, both arteries and veins.

They all cause reduced peripheral resistance (and therefore blood pressure) and pooling of blood in the periphery and, therefore, reduced venous return to the heart (preload).

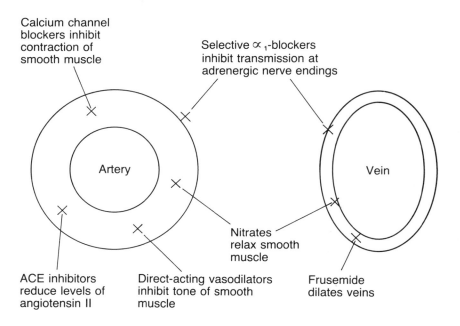

Figure 2.3F Action of vasodilators

They can be divided into six main groups, each of which will be treated in a separate section:

nitrates (e.g. GTN, ISMN)
calcium-channel blockers (e.g. nifedipine)
ACE inhibitors (e.g. captopril, enalapril)
adrenergic neurone-blocking drugs (e.g. guanethidine)
alpha-adrenoceptor-blocking drugs (e.g. prazosin)
direct-acting vasodilators (e.g. hydralazine).

NITRATES

How do they work?

They relax smooth muscle and cause dilatation of blood vessels and of the oesophagus. Their main effect is dilatation of the veins, which results in pooling of blood in the periphery and reduction of venous return to the heart (preload). This causes a rapid reduction in cardiac work load, which is why they are so useful in angina. The arterial dilatation is less pronounced but does improve coronary flow to a significant extent.

Who should take them?

Angina is the main indication, but they are also useful in the early stages of acute myocardial infarction and acute left ventricular failure.

Who should not take them?

There are no contra-indications but side-effects are common and some people cannot tolerate them. Side-effects include headache, postural hypotension, flushing and tachycardia.

Which preparation?

Glyceryl trinitrate is available in several different forms:
- tablets to be taken sublingually: 300; 500; 600 mcg;
- aerosol spray to be used in the mouth: 400 mcg/dose
(must not be shaken before use);
- slow-release tablet: sublingual or swallowed: various strengths;
- ointment: 1 inch (2.5 cm) contains 16.64 mg;
- impregnated plaster: 5 mg in 24 h.

Isosorbide dinitrate tablets (ISDN):
  – 5 mg; 10 mg: sublingually or swallowed.

Isosorbide mononitrate tablets (ISMN):
  – 10 mg; 20 mg: swallowed.

What dose?

See Angina (p.165).

What problems?

Side-effects can often be avoided if a small dose is used to start with. Another trick is to suggest the patient spits out the remainder of a sublingual preparation once it has started to have an effect but before the headache develops.

Tolerance reduces side-effects after a while but also results in a lessening of the desired effect. It may be avoided by building a nitrate-free period into every day. Preparations which attempt to provide continuous blood levels over 24 h may not be a good idea.

Storage: the shelf-life of GTN tablets is limited to 3 months after the bottle has been opened. This may be reduced if they are kept in a warm place like a trouser pocket but they are not much use to the patient if they are kept in the fridge at home! Other preparations are more stable.

Interactions with other drugs

There are no true interactions but, if given with other vasodilator or hypotensive drugs, postural hypotension may be a problem.

POINTS

With nitrates:

  – start with a low dose to avoid headache

  – avoid tolerance by including a daily drug-free period

  – remember the short shelf life of GTN tablets

  – use GTN before activity as well as for pain

CALCIUM-CHANNEL BLOCKING DRUGS

What are they?

The drugs in this group are chemically dissimilar and this is reflected in their widely differing modes of action and clinical applications.

How do they work?

They interfere with the movement of calcium ions across cell membranes. The effect of this is to reduce the activity of the cell. In the myocardium, this reduces contractility and excitability. Smooth muscle tone is reduced, peripheral arterioles dilate and peripheral resistance falls.

Calcium antagonists are therefore not simply vasodilators. They have three different types of effect on the cardiovascular system, although each drug within the group has a different spectrum of activity (Table 2.3B).

(1)   The reduced myocardial contractility (negative inotropism) causes reduced cardiac output, work load and oxygen requirements. This effect is balanced by the reduction in afterload resulting from peripheral vasodilatation so that the risk of heart failure is less than that seen with beta-blockers.

(2)   The antiarrhythmic action results from delayed A–V nodal conduction (especially verapamil). This is helpful in supra-ventricular tachycardias; dangerous in heart block.

(3)   Arteriolar vasodilatation causes dilatation of the coronary arteries, a fall in peripheral resistance, blood pressure and afterload.

This group of drugs is useful in:

-   angina because they reduce after-load, myocardial oxygen demand and increase coronary blood flow;

-   hypertension because they reduce peripheral resistance;

-   supra-ventricular tachycardias because they delay A–V nodal conduction;

-   patients who also have peripheral vascular disease.

Table 2.3B Actions of calcium-channel blocking drugs

	Reduced myocardial contractility	Reduced conduction through A – V node	Vasodilation	Oral dose
Nifedipine (Adalat)	0	0	+ + +	10 – 20 mg three times a d.
Verapamil (Cordilox)	+ +	+ +	+	40 – 120 mg onc daily increasing three times a d.
Diltiazem (Tildiem)	+	+	+	60 – 120 mg thre times a day
Nicardipine (Cardene)	0	0	+ +	20 – 30 mg three times a day
Clinical indications	Hypertension (care in heart failure)	SVT (care in conduction defects)	Angina Hypertension Raynaud's phenomenon	

Who should take them?

All the drugs in this group are effective in the treatment of angina and hypertension. Diltiazems and verapamil are pharmacologically similar. They are especially effective in SVT, but caution is needed if they are combined with beta-blockers because of the risk of extreme bradycardia. Nifedipine can be used safely with beta-blockers; nicardipine is least likely to depress contractility and cause dangerous reduction in cardiac output in a patient in whom there is a risk of heart failure.

Who should not take them?

Verapamil and diltiazem should not be given to patients with:
  bradycardia
  delayed conduction.
  heart failure.
Apart from aortic stenosis, there are no absolute contra-indications to the other members of the group but they may exacerbate hypotension if used in conjunction with nitrates and/or beta-blockers.

Side-effects

These are all usually minor and include:
     headache and flushing, especially early in treatment
     lethargy
     dependent oedema
     constipation (verapamil)
     nausea (diltiazem).

Interactions with other drugs

Verapamil can cause serious side-effects, if taken with:
     beta-blockers
     digoxin
     prazosin
     quinidine
     disopyramide

However, it is sometimes used in these combinations by cardiologists, under careful supervision.

POINTS

Calcium-channel blocking drugs are useful:

– in treatment of hypertension and angina

– when beta-blockers are contraindicated by asthma or PVD

– combined with beta-blockers (nifedipine)

– add to the risk of heart failure when used with beta-blockers

---

ANGIOTENSIN-CONVERTING ENZYME (ACE) INHIBITORS

How do they work?

As their name implies, they inhibit the action of angiotensin-converting enzyme and therefore interrupt the chain reaction leading to the formation of angiotensin II and aldosterone (see Figure 1.3H). By preventing the formation of angiotensin II, ACE inhibitors block the vasoconstrictor and sodium- and water-retaining effects of this system.

Therefore, ACE inhibitors reduce peripheral resistance and reduce blood pressure; limit fluid retention and act as mild potassium-sparing diuretics. They also act as venodilators, thus reducing venous return to the right side of the heart and cardiac workload.

Who should take them?

At present, they are used only when better-established drugs fail, and in general practice are licensed only for the treatment of hypertension. They have recently been shown to have a significant effect in patients with moderate to severe heart failure but they have to be used with caution in anyone with electrolyte disturbance or renal failure. Patients with heart failure are usually admitted to hospital for initiation of treatment with ACE inhibitors.

Who should not take them?

They are contra-indicated in renal failure, renal artery stenosis and pregnancy.

Care is needed in patients with impaired renal function and those taking potassium-sparing diuretics, especially spironolactone, which is itself an aldosterone antagonist.

What dose?

The initial dose should be half of the minimum dose (see Side-effects, below).

Hypertension: captopril: 12.5 mg to 50 mg (max) twice daily
enalapril: 5 mg to 40 mg (max) twice daily.
Heart failure: captopril: starting 6.25 mg three times daily
enalapril: starting 2.5 mg twice daily

Side-effects

There is a risk of hypotension with the first dose and it is therefore usual to start with a very small dose (e.g. 2.5 mg of enalapril or 6.25 mg captopril), taken in the evening, lying down.

The following may occur:

dry cough	proteinuria
loss of taste	neutropaenia, agranulocytosis
stomatitis	hyperkalaemia
rashes, angioedema	deteriorating renal function.

What precautions should you take?

Side-effects may be avoided by:

(1)   using a test dose;
(2)   keeping the dose as low as possible;
(3)   taking blood for urea and electrolytes before starting treatment and at regular intervals after: daily in heart failure to start with;
(4)   avoiding use with potassium-sparing diuretics and potassium supplements.

Interactions with other drugs

Diuretics: it is easy to produce hypotension and oliguria in patients already taking diuretics, who are likely to have electrolyte depletion. However, in hypertension the action of ACE inhibitors is usefully enhanced by modest sodium depletion, often achieved with low-dose diuretics.

Potassium-sparing diuretics, especialy spironolactone, should not be given with ACE inhibitors because of the risk of hyperkalaemia.

POINTS

In ACE inhibitor therapy:

– daily supervision is needed when initiating treatment in heart failure

– blood urea must be known and monitored

– watch for hyperkalaemia: avoid potassium-sparing diuretics

ADRENERGIC NEURONE-BLOCKING DRUGS

This is a group of drugs, which includes guanethidine, which block neurotransmission at the sympathetic ganglia. They have both alpha- and beta-blocking effects (see Figure 1.3I, p.18). Peripheral vasodilatation predominates, causing postural hypotension. For this reason, they have been replaced by better drugs.

ALPHA-ADRENOCEPTOR-BLOCKING DRUGS

What are they?

A group of drugs which block the alpha-receptors in the smooth muscle of arterioles (see Figure 1.3I).

How do they work?

The receptors are of two types, $alpha_1$ and $alpha_2$:

(1) $Alpha_1$ receptors facilitate vasoconstriction; blocking of these causes vasodilatation, reduced peripheral resistance and reduced blood pressure.

(2) $Alpha_2$ receptors inhibit local release of noradrenaline; blocking of these leads to an increase in circulating noradrenaline, which increases heart rate and contractility. This increases the blood pressure by increasing cardiac output.

If both receptors are inhibited, there may be little overall benefit. The first drugs in this group to be developed were non-specific and blocked both types of receptor (e.g. phentolamine).

The latest, such as prazosin and terazosin, are selective $alpha_1$ blocking drugs and may prove to be more successful.

Who should take them?

These are effective hypotensive drugs but, since they are relatively new, they are at present being used only when other treatment is contra-indicated or unsuccessful.

Who should not take them?

There are no recognised contra-indications at present.

What dose?

First-dose syncope may occur and so the drug should be introduced gradually
and given at night. A plan for starting prazosin might be:
- 1st week: 1 mg at night;
- 2nd week: 1 mg in the morning; 1 mg at night;
- increase at this rate until hypertension is controlled;
- maximum dose: 20 mg daily, divided into 2 or 3 doses.

Side-effects

Apart from first-dose syncope, none have yet been reported.
They appear to have no adverse effects on lipids.

POINT

With alpha-adrenoceptor-blocking drugs:

- start with a small dose at night

DIRECT-ACTING VASODILATORS

What are they?

Drugs which have a direct effect on the smooth muscle of arterioles (e.g. hydralazine).

Who should take hydralazine?

It is an effective hypotensive drug but is reserved for patients with particular problems because it can cause systemic lupus erythematosus (see below).

It is useful in patients with impaired renal function or hypertension resistant to other treat.nent. It improves renal blood flow but causes sodium retention.

What dose?

25 mg twice daily increasing to a maximum of 50 mg twice daily.

What problems?

Hydralazine may cause systemic lupus erythematosus, especially in women and if given in large doses. The dose should be limited to a maximum of 100 mg daily. It is best used in conjunction with a beta-blocker because it tends to cause reflex tachycardia if used alone.

POINTS

In hydralazine therapy:

- watch for SLE, especially in women

- maximum dose 100 mg daily

- postural hypotension may occur

ANTI-ARRHYTHMIC DRUGS

What are they?

A number of different drugs are used for the treatment of arrhythmias (see Table 2.3C). Several have already been described: beta-blockers (see p.59), calcium-channel blockers (e.g. verapamil; see p.69) and digoxin (see p.47). Amiodarone and disopyramide are described here.

What does amiodarone do?

Delays repolarisation and so increases refractory period.

Who should take it?

The main indication is the Wolff – Parkinson – White syndrome.

It is used in other arrhythmias only if all else fails, as it has unpleasant side-effects, which include liver damage, photosensitivity, thyroid function problems, skin discolouration, lung damage and insomnia. Its use is only likely to be initiated by a cardiologist.

What precautions?

Anyone taking long-term amiodarone should have regular liver function tests, thyroid function tests and chest X-rays. Exposure to light should be avoided as much as possible. Interactions with other drugs may be a problem (see *BNF*).

POINT

With amiodarone therapy:

- side-effects may cause problems with liver, thyroid, lung, skin, insomnia

---

What does disopyramide do?

It slows depolarisation, increases the refractory period and decreases excitability of myocardium.

Who should take it?

Its main use is in ventricular arrhythmias, especially after myocardial infarction.

What precautions are necessary?

Disopyramide may exacerbate heart failure by depressing cardiac output. It has anticholinergic effects and should be avoided in patients with glaucoma or a tendency to retention of urine.

POINTS

With disopyramide therapy:

– watch for heart failure

– retention of urine may occur

– check for glaucoma

Table 2.3C Sites of action of antiarrhythmic drugs

	S–A node	A–V node	Anomalous pathways	Ventricular muscle
Digoxin	+	+ +	–	–
Beta-blockers	+	+	–	–
Amiodarone	+	–	+	+
Quinidine	+	–	+	+
Verapamil	+	+ +	–	–
Procaineamide	+	–	+	+
Disopyramide	+	–	+	+
Lignocaine	–	–	–	+ +
Tocainide	–	–	–	+
Mexiletine	–	–	–	+

ANTI-CLOTTING AGENTS

What are they?

These are a group of drugs which inhibit the clotting mechanism (see Figure 2.3G). They include warfarin, phenindione, heparin and aspirin. Fibrinolytic agents are now being introduced to disperse recently formed thrombi.

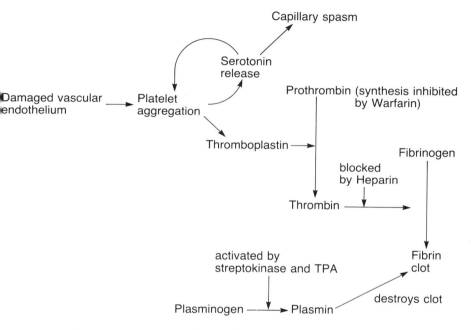

Figure 2.3G The clotting mechanism (simplified)

What do they do?

Warfarin, phenindione and heparin are true anticoagulants and reduce the tendency of clots to form in blood vessels, including the heart. Aspirin reduces the aggregation and stickiness of platelets.

How do they work?

(1)   Warfarin and phenindione inhibit the formation of prothrombin.
(2)   Aspirin inhibits thromboxane, a prostaglandin which activates platelets.
(3)   Heparin inhibits the action of thromboplastin.

79

Who should take them?

(1)   Warfarin is used to prevent the formation of thrombi within the heart and other blood vessels in patients at risk. These include patients with:

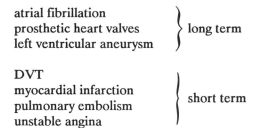

atrial fibrillation
prosthetic heart valves   } long term
left ventricular aneurysm

DVT
myocardial infarction   } short term
pulmonary embolism
unstable angina

Phenindione is used only if the patient is sensitive to warfarin.

(2)   Aspirin should be taken by everyone with ischaemic heart disease who is not taking warfarin.

(3)   Heparin is given to all patients admitted to hospital with myocardial infarction. It is not used in patients treated at home.

Who should not take them?

(1)   Warfarin should not be taken by patients with a bleeding tendency (e.g. haemophilia, thrombocytopaenia), active peptic ulceration, pericarditis, or pregnancy.

(2)   Aspirin should not be taken by patients taking warfarin because of the risk of bleeding.

Warfarin: what regime?

Warfarin is usually initiated in hospital:
   –   take blood for prothrombin time before the first dose;
   –   loading dose of 10 mg daily for three days;
            (reduced in frail people or liver disease);
   –   repeat prothrombin time on third day;
   –   dose thereafter regulated by prothrombin time:
            international normalised ratio (INR) kept between
            2 and 4.5, the higher levels for those at greatest risk.

CAMEO

Mary Horner is 36. She was found to have mitral stenosis during her second pregnancy, 8 years ago. She developed atrial fibrillation 3 years ago and has been on warfarin since then. Her husband is an engineer and when he was offered a job abroad, she went with him. Her prothrombin time and warfarin dose was supervised at a private clinic but after 3 months, she lost suddenly most of the sight of her left eye and was found to have had a retinal embolus. She returned to the UK and, with meticulous attention to her prothrombin time, has had no further problems.

Drug interactions with warfarin

These are numerous (see *BNF* for complete list) and occur with foods as well as drugs. Patients taking warfarin should be given an advice sheet about the precautions they should take and the food and drugs to avoid.

Warfarin is carried bound to proteins in the blood stream and it is broken down by the liver. Any substance which dislodges it from its binding sites, increases its effect. Any substance which induces liver enzymes increases the rate of breakdown of the drug and reduces its effect. As long as these drugs are taken regularly, the effect is reflected in the prothrombin time and the dose of warfarin adjusted accordingly.

Bleeding in patients taking warfarin

(1)   Stop the drug.
(2)   Give vitamin K (Konakion): 10 mg i.v. SLOWLY.
(3)   Consider admission to hospital.

Table 2.3D Modification of warfarin effects by other drugs

Reduced by	Increased by
Carbamazipine	Alcohol
Barbiturates	Sulphonamides
Phenytoin	Cimetidine
Oral contraceptives	Amiodarone
Vitamin K	Clofibrate
	Metronidazole

Fibrinolytic drugs are not yet generally available

Three drugs in this group are at present in use: streptokinase, tissue plasminogen activator (TPA) and anysolated plasminogen streptokinase activator compound (APSAC). They are used in acute myocardial infarction to disperse the clot, which has formed in the coronary artery. They are given intravenously as soon as possible after the infarction has occurred, streptokinase and TPA by continuous infusion; APSAC by a single slow injection. A reduction in mortality of 40% has been reported.

POINTS

With anti-clotting agents:

- prothrombin time and warfarin dose need regular monitoring

- drug interactions with warfarin are common

- aspirin is useful prevention after ischaemic events

PART 3:
THE DIAGNOSTIC
PROCESS

3.1
Introduction

The clinical history, examination and investigations form the basis of the diagnostic process.

Medical students are taught to gather all the information they can, before considering what might be wrong with the patient. Experienced doctors draw up a short list of possible diagnoses at an early stage in the consultation and repeatedly review and revise it as the diagnostic process proceeds. The list is refined, some hypotheses being excluded, while others are placed higher in the list until a single probable diagnosis is reached or at least the serious possibilities are excluded. Initially, the list may contain pathophysiological states, such as heart failure or angina, rather than diseases, such as hypertension or ischaemic heart disease. If one of these, say heart failure, is confirmed, then the process of refinement continues until the underlying disease, perhaps hypertension, and the precipitating cause, myocardial infarction, are both identified.

The diagnostic process does not stop until the diagnosis is as complete as it needs to be in the circumstances. How complete it needs to be depends on a number of factors, including the age of the patient, the presence of other disease and the treatment options available. For instance, if the pathophysiological state, diagnosed at a very early stage, is 'tachyarrhythmia' and the patient is young and fit and little troubled by symptoms, it would be quite proper to leave the diagnostic process at this stage. No treatment is needed and further elucidation is unnecessary. If the pathophysiological state is heart failure, it may be due to mitral stenosis with the recent onset of atrial fibrillation as the precipitating cause. Treatment with digoxin, anticoagulants and mitral valve replacement may be needed. The patient is deprived of these if the diagnostic process stops at heart failure.

The chapters in Part 3 consist of:

Chapter 3.2: Clinical History;
Chapter 3.3: Sorting Out the Symptoms;
Chapter 3.4: Examination;
Chapter 3.5: Electrocardiology;
Chapter 3.6: Pathological Tests and Chest X-rays.

These are the elements of the diagnostic process; the clinical history, examination and investigations are all investigative tools, which should be used, selectively and economically, when needed. At any time, the decision as to what to do next depends on the information so far revealed and the current list of possible diagnoses. The process may be completed in a few minutes or extended over a long period. There is often no reason to hurry. Time itself is a valuable aid to diagnosis.

THE AIMS OF THE DIAGNOSTIC PROCESS

The diagnostic process has two main aims:

(1)   Early, accurate diagnosis of symptomatic disease.
         To achieve the first aim, a search is made for clues which might point, on the one hand to a healthy heart, or, on the other, to disease.
         This includes having a high index of suspicion of heart disease when faced with common symptoms. For instance cough and wheeze (is it asthma or left ventricular failure?) and dizzy spells, which could be the familiar, undiagnosable non-disease or potentially fatal (but eminently treatable) heart block.

(2)   Identification of treatable disease at an early stage, before it has caused symptoms (secondary prevention).
         To achieve the second aim, screening of some sort has to be undertaken. It can be mass, selective or opportunistic (see p.317). The history will suggest who should be especially sought out for further attention.
         The prime example of this is hypertension. Others are hyperlipidaemia and aortic stenosis.

3.2
Clinical History

Is there anything to suggest cardiovascular disease?

- *family history*: ischaemic heart disease, hypertension;

- *previous medical history*: rheumatic fever, hypertension, myocardial infarction;

- *previous medical findings*: normal and abnormal;

- *present state of fitness*: exercise tolerance, well-being;

- *symptoms*: presented by the patient; discovered by the doctor.

The history can provide more useful information than any other clinical tool and it is worth taking trouble to make it accurate and complete. The main problems are that it takes so long and that it has to be repeated every time the patient is seen.

The great advantage of general practice is that many patients remain registered with the same practice for a long time. Even if they move away, their records (unlike hospital records) follow them. It is a simple matter to keep a continuous running history, on a summary card or front sheet, during the patient's time with the practice. There is no good reason why it should not be kept up throughout life: the patient might keep a copy so that it stayed with him wherever he went. If this is done, then all that is needed, when the patient attends with a new complaint, is to check that it is up to date, fill in any gaps and concentrate on the present problem. The basic information does not even have to be collected and entered by a doctor. If a nurse sees the patient on first registering or for routine health checks at regular intervals, he or she enters the data. It can be updated by any member of the practice team, according to an agreed protocol, whenever any event affects the patient or his family.

The basic data

Family history

– Date, age and cause of death of all first-degree relatives (parents, siblings, children).

– Any relevant disease in first-degree relatives.

Personal history

Domestic situation/ sources of stress
Occupation: any particular risks
Smoking: never/ex/current (amount)
Alcohol
Addictive drugs
Sport/ hobbies
Literate or not.

Previous medical history

Serious diseases at any age
Operations
Confinements
Routine medicals with dates and recordings of BP, abnormal clinical findings, weight
Test results with dates: ECG, chest X-ray, cervical smear, etc.
Hospital referrals: current, previous.

Medication

Previous significant medication
Current medication: name of drugs and doses
Drug sensitivities.

Immunisations

Details and dates with reactions, if any.

Allergies and drug sensitivities

Only important reactions need be recorded.

This is a massive amount of information but it can be compressed and tabulated to take up very little space. Over all, space is saved, as well as time, because these facts never have to be recorded again anywhere else. Such a system makes dangerous mistakes easier to avoid and may be a protection in case of legal problems.

Risk factors

Systematic record keeping enables patients at special risk of heart disease to be identified. The notes can be flagged with a warning sticker.
Significant factors are:

  Male sex
  Age over 40
  Family history of   – ischaemic heart disease under 65
                        – hypertension
                        – diabetes

  Hyperlipidaemia
  Smoking
  Obesity
  Diabetes
  Hypertension
  Alcohol abuse
  High stress
  Unhealthy diet.

WHAT IS THE PRESENT COMPLAINT?

Whatever the initial symptom presented, specific enquiry should be made for all other symptoms which might indicate cardiovascular or other relevant disease. Patients cannot be relied upon to tell the doctor all the relevant facts. Sometimes they feel they must ration the number of things they complain about in case the doctor thinks they are moaners. Sometimes they simply do not realise that something is significant. Sometimes, what the doctor needs to know is that the patient does not have a particular problem.

Why has the patient come about it now?

Is it new, worse or beginning to worry him? Has something happened, like the sudden death of a friend or relative, to make him uneasy about himself? What does he think it might be? Doctors often reassure people that they have not got some disease which they never thought they had and fail to recognise that they are worried about another, which the doctor had not considered as a possibility. For example many people with dizzy turns think they are about to have a stroke.

CAMEO

Eileen Saunders is 52. She is an anxious woman with a quiet, diffident manner. She visits her doctor complaining of dizzy feelings, during which she becomes breathless and has pins and needles and a tight feeling in her hands. The doctor examines her and diagnoses hyperventilation. He tries to explain what is causing the attacks. She thanks him and leaves the consulting room.

On the way out, she meets the nurse who looked after her husband during his last illness about a year before.

'Hello, Eileen. How are you?'

'I am not at all well, nurse. I keep having these turns and they frighten me. You know my mother died of a stroke at my age.'

The nurse arranges for her to return to explain her fears to the doctor, who is able to reassure her completely.

89

3.3
Sorting Out the Symptoms

Any symptom can be due to serious disease. The symptoms which can indicate cardiovascular disease are many and varied, from tiredness to chest pain, swollen feet to breathlessness. All these symptoms are common in completely healthy people and in others with diseases of other systems.

Whenever a doctor is faced with a patient with a symptom, he or she is continuously considering whether this particular symptom, in this patient, is likely to be due to 'anything serious'.

This assessment starts as soon as the patient enters the room, sometimes before. It is based partly on a knowledge of probabilities: the incidence of disease in regard to age and sex and situation. It also involves recognising whether and how much this individual's physiological processes are being disturbed: does he 'look well'? Are there other indicators of disease?

If the patient is a bright, healthy-looking 24-year-old woman, ischaemic heart disease will not be very high on the list of possible causes of her chest pain.

This ordering of differential diagnoses is, for the most part, an unconscious process. It is done without thinking. This is no bad thing as it saves time and makes for increased efficiency. It stops us chasing, unnecessarily, after unlikely diagnoses.

However, the unconsciousness of the process carries risks. It becomes safe and effective only with experience; experience is selective and there may be gaps, of which the doctor is not aware; this allows him or her not to consider diagnoses, which should be considered but which simply do not spring to mind. It is difficult constantly to consider unusual but important possibilities which are not seen very often. Therefore, it can be useful to review and refresh the way in which these very rapid assessments are made.

Throughout this book we draw attention to the incidence of cardiac pathology: who gets what and when?

In this chapter, we look at symptoms with particular emphasis on the presence of physiological disturbance, which should alert the doctor to the possibility of serious disease.

We will consider:

In each of these, age, sex, lifestyle and previous knowledge of the patient can provide vital clues. History of previous illnesses and family history are important. It is also useful to enquire whether the patient has had previous episodes of a similar nature.

CHEST PAIN

Chest pain is one of the commonest symptoms: it worries both patients and doctors because both know that, although it is usually insignificant, it can be imminently life-threatening and recognising it may make a difference to the outcome. It can be extremely difficult to elucidate and what follows can only provide some general guidelines. Cardiac ischaemia can be completely painless; it can cause devastatingly severe pain; it can cause anything between. It is frequently atypical, occurring at rest and not on exercise, or inconsistent, behaving differently at different times.

What might it be?

(1)   Cardiovascular causes:
     − ischaemic pain: angina; myocardial infarction
     − pericarditis
     − dissecting aneurysm
     − pulmonary embolism.
(2)   Non-cardiovascular causes:
     − lung disease
     − gastrointestinal disease
     − musculoskeletal problems
     − herpes zoster.

How does he look and feel?

Does he look?
   Ill
   Pale
   Sweaty
   Breathless
   In pain
   Febrile
   Frightened
   Talking easily
   Fit and well.

Does he feel?
   In pain now
   Faint, dizzy
   Breathless
   Feverish
   Frightened
   Calm and relaxed.

Where is the pain?

Central	*To one side*
Myocardial ischaemia	Pleurisy
infarction	Herpes zoster
angina	Musculoskeletal
Dissecting aneurysm	Texidor's twinge
Pericarditis	Bornholm's disease
Dyspepsia	Metastases
Musculoskeletal	Cardiac neurosis
Cardiac neurosis	Peripheral pulmonary embolism.
Massive pulmonary embolism.	

What is the pain like?

Ischaemic pain	*Non-ischaemic pain*
Severe	Aching
Crushing	Variable
Heavy: 'like a weight'	Sharp
Tight	Dull
Constricting: 'like a band'.	Superficial
	Pleuritic.

Watch for non-verbal signals: the clenched fist, held against the sternum, often accompanies the description of ischaemic pain.

Where does it go?

Ischaemic pain may radiate or be confined to neck, jaw, upper limbs, back.
   Oesophageal pain may radiate in a similar way.

How long does it last?

< 5 Minutes	*5 – 15 Minutes*	*Continuous*
Angina.	Dyspepsia	Musculoskeletal
	Angina	Myocardial infarction
	Musculoskeletal.	Dissecting aneurysm
		Herpes zoster
		Pericarditis
		Pulmonary embolism.

What brings it on?

Exertion	*Food*	*Movement*	*Respiration*
Angina.	Dyspepsia Angina.	Musculoskeletal.	Pleurisy Pericarditis.

What relieves it?

Rest	*GTN*	*Antacids*	*Analgesics*	*Change of position*
Angina.	Angina Oesophageal spasm Musculoskeletal.	Dyspepsia.	Musculoskeletal Herpes zoster Pericarditis Pleurisy.	Musculoskeletal Pericarditis.

Are there any other symptoms?

Palpitations	Fatigue
Breathlessness	Reduced exercise tolerance
Oedema	Cough
Dizzy spells	Nausea
Blackouts	Vomiting
Fever.	

CAMEO

Brian Harris was 52, a very intense, self-employed builder. He was once a successful sportsman and helped with the local athletics club. He had gone to seed rather spectacularly and was overweight and smoked and drank fairly heavily. He visited his doctor regularly over a period of about 2 years complaining of epigastric and retrosternal pain. It occurred at any time but especially after meals. It tended to last about 10–15 min but he had a persistent discomfort most of the time. It was relieved by antacids and by belching.

Examination revealed nothing apart from his general unhealthy aspect. His ECG was unremarkable and a barium swallow was reported as showing oesophageal reflux. He was treated with antacids and general advice about his life style and felt better.

He came into the surgery on a Saturday morning, having had persistent pain, of the same kind as before, for 2 hours. He was on his way on holiday, towing a caravan. There were no new physical signs. An ECG was the same as the last one, 6 weeks ago. The doctor felt uneasy but reassured him and sent him on his way.

Later that day, he collapsed and died, while setting up the caravan. The post mortem revealed a large, fresh myocardial infarct and several small, old ones with extensive, severe coronary artery disease.

BREATHLESSNESS

This is another common symptom, often elicited by questions from the doctor rather than presented as the primary complaint. It can, sometimes, be difficult to discover whether the patient is in fact abnormally breathless or merely unfit. It can be made easier by the rest of the history and by the doctor's previous knowledge of the patient. Breathlessness should be thought of as falling into two distinct categories, each of which will be considered independently: the acute (continuing) attack and intermittent attacks.

Acute (continuing) attack of breathlessness

Possible causes:

Bronchial asthma	Pulmonary embolism
Left heart failure	Pneumonia
Pneumothorax	Acute bronchitis.
Hysterical hyperventilation	

How does he look and feel?

Does he look?
Ill
Pale
Cyanosed
Distressed
Breathless
Coughing
Talking easily
Fit and well.

Does he feel?
Breathless now
Feverish
Anxious
Chest pain.

When/how did it start?

Did it start suddenly or develop gradually over a period of time? Did something trigger the attack (e.g. allergy, URTI)? Have there been any other symptoms such as chest pain, fever, cough, palpitations? Has it happened before?

Intermittent attacks of breathlessness

Possible causes:
    Bronchial asthma
    Left heart failure
    Carcinoma of lung
    Hysterical hyperventilation
    Chronic bronchitis/emphysema.

The most important distinction to be made is between left heart failure and bronchial asthma.

When does it occur?

Left heart failure
    On exercise
    On lying down
    At night.

Bronchial asthma
    On exercise
    Exposure to allergens
    In smoky atmosphere
    At night.

What relieves it?

Left heart failure
    Resting
    Sitting up
    GTN.

Bronchial asthma
    Bronchodilator inhaler.

Are there any other symptoms?

    Chest pain
    Cough
    Haemoptysis
    Peripheral oedema
    Leg pain or swelling.

CAMEO

Samuel Hampton, aged 52, was a new patient to the practice. A fat, flamboyant, plethoric character, he had been treated with atenolol and nifedipine for hypertension. He had become increasingly breathless for the last week and had been given antibiotics, without improvement. He admitted that the breathlessness was worse at night and that he had woken, fighting for breath, on two occasions in the small hours.

He weighed 18 stone and his blood pressure was 210/120, using the large cuff; pulse, 80 per minute, regular. There were scattered rhonchi throughout both lung fields with crepitations at the right base. A chest X-ray confirmed pulmonary venous congestion.

PALPITATIONS

The problem with this symptom is that there is no universally agreed definition of what it means. Even doctors disagree in defining the term.

A common experience is:
Doctor: 'Do you suffer from palpitations?'
Patient: 'No.'
Doctor: 'Do you know what palpitations are?'
Patient: 'No.'
Doctor: 'Palpitations is being aware of your heart beating.'
Patient: 'Oh, I often get that.'

We will use the following definition:
Palpitations are felt when the patient is aware of his or her heart beating in an abnormal way.

The sensation may be one which would be normal under certain circumstances, such as after running for a bus, but not normal at rest. It may also be one which is in itself abnormal, such as a completely irregular heart beat or one which is much faster than it would ever normally be.

What might it be?

- A heightened awareness of the normal heart beat (e.g. due to fear or anxiety);
- Extrasystoles;
- Sinus tachycardia (e.g. due to hyperthyroidism or anxiety);
- Paroxysmal supraventricular tachycardia;
- Atrial fibrillation;
- Atrial flutter;
- Ventricular tachycardia.

Which is it?

Repeated attacks

The diagnosis can often be made from listening carefully to the description the patient gives. You need to know:

− How long do the attacks last?
    − a single beat at a time
    − a few seconds
    − minutes/hours.

− How does it start?
    − suddenly
    − gradually.

− How does it stop?
    − suddenly
    − gradually.

− What exactly is it like?
    − fast/slow
    − regular/ irregular
    − most patients can tap it out on the desk fairly accurately.

− How do you feel during the attack?
    − awful: has to stop
    − OK: can continue
    − breathless
    − chest pain
    − faint/dizzy (lose consciousness?).

− When does it happen?
    − on exertion
    − at rest
    − in bed.

− What brings it on?
    − coffee, alcohol
    − stress
    − exercise.

− How often do you get it?

- How much does it affect you?

- Does anything stop the attack?
  - holding breath
  - rest.
- Do you know how fast your pulse is during an attack?

- What do you look like during an attack?
  - normal
  - pale
  - flushed.

CAMEO

Andrew Stanley was 42. He had suffered from palpitations since childhood. They had recently become more obtrusive. The attacks started suddenly at any time and usually lasted about 20 min although one or two had persisted for 3 – 4 hours. He felt a pounding in the chest and dizzyness, weakness and breathlessness. There was some precordial discomfort but no pain. He did not have to stop what he is doing but was more comfortable if he sat down until the attack wore off.

When asked to tap out the rhythm on his chest, he demonstrated a rapid regular rate of about 160 per min. A resting ECG was normal.

Giving up coffee reduced the frequency of the attacks and he found that dropping down sharply on one knee, as if to do up a shoe-lace, stopped the attacks immediately.

Continuing attack

Many of the questions above may be useful but clinical examination and ECG will immediately elucidate the problem.

Are there any symptoms between attacks such as:
   chest pain
   breathlessness
   dizzy spells
   faints?

Has there ever been an episode, such as loss of speech or weakness of a limb, which might suggest cerebral embolism?

PERIPHERAL OEDEMA: SWELLING OF BOTH FEET

What might it be?

- Imagination: it is amazing how many people interpret weight gain or the bloated, unfit sensation following a holiday as 'swelling'.

- Idiopathic: the most numerous; occurs in warm weather and when people are immobile, for instance when travelling or confined to a chair for some other reason. It is not due to fluid retention but associated with increased capillary permeability and venous stasis.
- Allergic reaction.

- Reduced serum albumen, e.g. nephrotic syndrome.

- Right heart failure, either alone or as part of congestive failure.

Once the presence of true oedema is confirmed, it may already be possible to make a firm diagnosis. If cardiac disease is a possibility, the usual questions about other symptoms should be asked.

FATIGUE

This is a universal symptom and one which most doctors dread. It is difficult to sort out and yet of potential significance, especially in cardiac disease.

An especially high index of suspicion of heart disease is needed in patients who are over 40 and:

> are male
> smoke
> have hypertension
> have family history of heart disease
> have a previous history suggestive of ischaemic heart disease
> have rheumatic heart disease.

What might it be?

Myocardial infarction	Anaemia
Pre-infarction syndrome	Sub-acute bacterial endocarditis
Arrhythmia	Drug toxicity
Heart failure	Other (non-cardiac) conditions.

Are there any other symptoms?

Chest pain   Palpitations
Breathlessness   Fever/night sweats
Oedema   Weight loss.

CAMEO

Elizabeth Sheffield comes to see the doctor complaining of feeling increasingly tired with multiple aches and pains during the last 6 months. She is 32 and has three young children and a disorganised husband. The doctor can find nothing to explain her symptom and puts it down to the stresses of family life.

During the next few weeks, she becomes worse and one morning she is so weak that she can hardly get out of bed. Her husband takes the day off to bring her to the surgery and she is weepy and miserable. She is clearly depressed but the degree of muscular weakness is impressive and amongst her many symptoms is central chest pain.

The doctor is puzzled and does a battery of tests including thyroid function tests and ECG. To his surprise, these show that she is hypothyroid and she recovers completely on replacement therapy.

DIZZY SPELLS AND FAINTING ATTACKS

What might they be?

(1) Cardiovascular causes:
         arrhythmias: bradycardia, ventricular tachycardia
         postural hypotension (?hypotensive drugs)
         transient ischaemic attacks
         cerebral emboli
         aortic stenosis
         heart failure.

(2) Non-cardiovascular causes:
         epilepsy
         vertigo
         simple faints (vaso-vagal attacks)
         hyperventilation
         hysteria/ neurosis
         fever.

What do you need to know?

- What are the attacks like?

- How long do they last?

- What brings on an attack?

- Do you have any other symptoms before, during or after the attacks?

- Do you feel yourself passing out?

- What do you look like during an attack?
    - pale
    - blue.

- Have you ever hurt yourself, passed urine or bitten your tongue during an attack?

- Is there any warning that the attack is coming?

- How do you feel afterwards?
    - sleepy
    - tired
    - normal.

3.4
Examination

In an ideal world, every patient would have a full physical examination on joining the practice and a useful baseline of observations would be available for future visits.

Few practices can manage this, although an increasing number of people have routine medicals for employment, sport or insurance purposes. The problem is that findings from these are seldom made available to the family doctor.

CAMEO

Ken Gore was 27. He was not registered with the practice but came for a routine medical for a private pilot's licence. His blood pressure was 150/105. He had never had it taken before. His femoral pulses were palpable but reduced in volume and delayed when compared with the radial pulse. A bruit was heard over the left scapula.

He was refused the licence and advised to see his GP.

A year later, he returned, having had an operation for coarctation of the aorta. His blood pressure was 118/72 and he was granted his licence.

Commonsense, as well as time constraints, dictate that it is neither possible nor desirable to conduct a full physical examination on every patient entering the consulting room. It is therefore necessary to decide which patient must be examined fully at once; which should be examined fully sometime; and which needs less than a full examination. In some patients it will be necessary to conduct a complete examination of every system in order to elucidate the problem but in most it is possible to be selective in the choice of procedures without risk of missing anything important.

Thus, if the patient is a fit young woman complaining of palpitations, which sound like supraventricular tachycardia, few experienced GPs will examine the foot pulses and the liver, though an ECG would be a good idea to exclude a short P – R interval, which might suggest W – P – W.

Within the general aims of the overall diagnostic process, the specific purpose of the examination is to help answer the following six questions.

(1)   *Is the patient in acute distress?*

    – There may be pain, breathlessness, confusion, collapse, unconsciousness.

    – If so, is the cause cardiovascular?

    – Are there signs of:
        – heart failure (see below)
        – myocardial infarction
        – arrhythmia
        – other CVS disorder?

(2)   *Is the cardiac output normal?*

    (a)   Reduced output:
        – There may be cold extremities, constricted veins, thready pulse, hypotension, confusion, dizzyness.

        – If so, are there signs of:
            – hypothyroidism
            – hypothermia
            – heart failure
            – other CVS disorder?

        – If signs of heart failure, are there signs of:
            – precipitating cause
            – underlying disease (see next section)?

    (b)   Increased output:
        – There may be hot extremities, dilated veins, bounding pulse.

        – If so, are there signs of:
            – hyperthyroidism
            – anaemia
            – fever
            – other CVS disorder?

(3)   *Is the venous pressure normal on both sides of the heart?*

    (a)   Increased on left: breathlessness
                          orthopnoea   } left heart failure
                          wet lung sounds

(b)   Increased on right: raised jugular venous pressure ⎱ right heart
                  (± oedema and hepatomegaly) ⎰ failure

(c)   If increased, are there signs of:

- precipitating cause of heart failure such as:
  - myocardial infarction
  - arrhythmia?

- underlying disease such as:
  - hypertension
  - valve disease
  - chronic lung disease
  - pulmonary embolism?

(4)   Is the heart beating normally?

(a)   *Pulse*: normal rate, shape, volume?

(b)   *Cardiac* impulse: normal?

- If not, is there evidence of:
  - reduced output
  - left ventricular hypertrophy (LVH)
  - right ventricular hypertrophy (RVH)
  - arrhythmia?

(5)   Are there signs of valve disease?

(a)   *Pulse*: may be, for example:
- collapsing (aortic regurgitation)
- slow rising (aortic stenosis).

(b)   *Individual chamber enlargement*: for example:
- LV+ in aortic valve disease
- RV+ in mitral stenosis.

(c)   *Extra sounds*: for example:
- an ejection click in aortic stenosis
- an opening snap in mitral stenosis.

(d)   *Murmurs*: for example:
  - apical diastolic in mitral stenosis
  - diamond-shaped systolic in aortic stenosis
  - early diastolic in aortic reguritation.

(6)   Is there anything to suggest ischaemic heart disease?

(a)   Atheroma:
  - xanthalasma
  - tendon xanthomata
  - arcus senilis.

(b)   Peripheral vascular disease:
  - foot pulses
  - carotid pulses.

For most GPs, there are three types of examination. In each, only signs which might be relevant are sought.

THREE TYPES OF EXAMINATION

Minimal examination

This consists of gaining as much information as possible from watching the patient as he enters the room and explains why he has come. A great deal can be gleaned from this, especially if the doctor already knows the patient well: Does he, or she, look well? – lively, vigorous, and of good colour? Did he move well on entering? – easily, without pain or stiffness? Is he breathless? – talking easily? Is he worried or frightened? Together with the history, these observations can provide a reasonable idea of gross cardiac function.

If the history is not particularly suggestive of cardiovascular disease and there is a recent record of the blood pressure, this may be all that is needed.

Intermediate examination

This consists of all the above plus as much as is possible without the patient being completely undressed and lying on a couch.

Only those items which are relevant are examined:

(1)   *Pulses*:
  - radial: rate and characteristics;

- foot: combined with observation of the peripheral perfusion and presence or absence of oedema;
- carotid:
  - are both present and equal?
  - are they normal?

(2) *Blood pressure*: try to avoid taking it as soon as the patient comes in, even if this is what he has come for. A more reliable baseline is obtained if it can be left until the last moment.

(3) *Heart*: can be examined very well, although incompletely, with the patient sitting, or standing, with shirt undone:
- heart size, type of cardiac impulse, sounds and most murmurs can be identified;
- however, the mitral diastolic murmur of mitral stenosis may not be heard in this position.

(4) *Lungs*: best examined standing up.

(5) *Optic fundi*: are best examined sitting or standing.

The main omissions from this list are the examination of the jugular venous pressure, liver, femoral pulses and abdomen.

However, this examination may be quite adequate for many situations, including many patients who are attending for follow-up or review of medication.

It is possible that elements in the history or signs observed in a minimal or intermediate examination will suggest the need for a full one.

Full examination

This is essential in two situations.

(1). Suspicion of heart failure or recent onset of another problem

The underlying cause and precipitating factor are being sought. Examples are:
breathlessness
peripheral oedema
angina
myocardial infarction
tachyarrhythmia
embolic event.

(2). *Abnormalities needing further elucidation*

If any abnormality, needing further elucidation, is found in the course of the history or previous examination then a full examination is needed. It does not necessarily always have to be done immediately and some doctors find it convenient to set aside time for 'long cases'.

CAMEO

Mary Power is 71. She came to see the doctor asking for 'something for bronchitis'. She had been increasingly breathless on exertion recently and had had two attacks of breathlessness, which had woken her at night.

She had a slow rising pulse, enlarged heart, left ventricular type of cardiac impulse and a loud aortic systolic murmur. Her ECG showed left ventricular hypertrophy (LVH). She was referred to a cardiologist with a diagnosis of aortic stenosis and her condition was considered sufficiently urgent to be given an aortic valve replacement within 3 weeks.

Experienced doctors each develop their own individual approach to clinical examination and, although this may need to be reviewed or sharpened up from time to time, it is not helpful to try to change it completely. It is not intended that this section should be used as a pattern for the clinical examination but rather as an *aide memoire*: a reminder of the most important points and those which are most likely to be forgotten or missed.

The order in which the various elements of the examination are carried out does not matter, but it is quicker and less likely that things will be left out if the same order is always used. It is also a good idea to leave auscultation until last and to have made as firm a short-list of differential diagnoses as possible before listening. The reason for this is that murmurs are often confusing and sometimes make an impression which is out of all proportion to their significance. "The heart is a pump, not a musical box", said Lord Brock, and how it functions is in fact more important than the noises it makes.

What should be written down

As much as possible should be recorded, especially negative findings. Medical shorthand is fine as long as it is legible: other doctors may need to refer to it.

A check list of what is important

(1)   *General appearance* (the feet must be uncovered)

        Young/old for age
        Lean; obese; cachectic
        Skin colour: cyanosis; pallor; plethora
        Skin temperature; peripheral veins; peripheral perfusion
        Xanthalasma; xanthomata (e.g. on tendons); arcus senilis
        Oedema (not cardiac unless JVP raised)
        Breathless; distressed; in pain
        Hands: clubbing; splinter haemorrhages; tremor.

(2)   *Blood pressure*

    – the inflatable part of the cuff should be over the front of the arm;

    – if the tubes get in the way, turn the cuff so that they come out of the top;

    – in some people, there is a silent period in the middle of the range, after the first sounds appear, so it is important to inflate the cuff well above the systolic pressure – if in doubt, check by palpation;
    – deflate slowly or a false reading may be obtained;

    – the diastolic pressure is taken from the 5th phase, i.e. when the sounds disappear;

    – take both sitting and standing, if postural hypotension is likely (elderly, drugs);

    – take at least twice, if raised.

(3)   *Pulses*

    – radial:
        – rate (remember apex rate may be different) – if irregular, does it vary with respiration?
        – volume: full; thready
        – characteristics: collapsing; slow rising
        – are they both the same?

    – foot: often difficult to feel (make a note if not found);

- femorals: is timing same as radial?

- carotids: present; equal; normal.

(4) *Jugular venous pressure*: measured in cm above the sternal angle in the internal jugular vein. If the person lies at 45°, the veins should not be seen to be filled above the clavicle. The external jugular vein is sometimes full, even in the upright position and is of no significance.

(5) *Heart*: quiet; hyperdynamic.

- Impulse: visible; palpable – hyperactivity, ventricular enlargement.

- Apex beat: normally found in the 4th intercostal space, in the mid-clavicular line. It is often difficult to feel (note if it is not found).

- Abnormal pulsations or thrills.

- *Auscultation*: use the bell of the stethoscope for low-pitched sounds (3rd and 4th) and mitral diastolic murmurs; the diaphragm for the 1st and 2nd sounds, opening snap, ejection clicks and aortic diastolic murmurs. Listen for one thing at a time.

  - Is the apex rate the same as the radial?

  - Are the sounds normal in number? (see also under Physiology p.29)

  - split sounds: the second heart sound is normally split but varies with respiration and is not 'fixed'. (The second component of the split is the closure of the pulmonary valve and is best heard in pulmonary area.)

  - if more than two, what is the timing of the extra sound (feel carotid while listening)?

  - extra sounds: *The 3rd heart sound* occurs just after the 2nd sound, early in diastole. It is sometimes called protodiastolic.
    The 4th heart sound is late in diastole, just before the 1st sound. It is sometimes called pre-systolic.
    Both 3rd and 4th heart sounds can be heard in normal people but are also associated with heart failure, when they cause a gallop rhythm.

An ejection click follows the first sound. It is usually associated with dilatation of the ascending aorta and is heard in the aortic area and at the apex.

An opening snap follows the second sound. It is usually due to mitral stenosis and may be the only physical sign. It is high-pitched, short and heard at the apex and even better at the left sternal edge.

– Are the sounds normal in intensity (relative to each other)? They are normally consistent from one beat to another but will vary from beat to beat if the rate or coordination varies, as when there are extrasystoles.

– *Murmurs*:
   – do not hurry.
   – listen to systole in each area, sitting.
   – listen to diastole in each area, sitting.

   – listen to the apex and around it with the patient lying on left side for mitral diastolic murmur.
   – listen to lower sternal area, with the patient holding breath out and leaning forward, for aortic diastolic murmur. Aortic systolic murmurs are also well heard using this manoevre.

– timing (may be difficult) – find where the murmur is loudest and then time it with carotid pulse.

– diastolic murmurs are always significant, systolic murmurs may or may not be.

– draw what you hear.

– systolic murmurs are common and often of no pathological significance. They occur in patients with increased output: pregnancy, childhood, fever, anaemia, hyperthyroidism.

– a systolic murmur is likely to be abnormal if:
   – it is accompanied by a thrill
   – it obliterates the second sound
   – it is widely conducted
   – it does not vary with the position of the patient
   – it is associated with a diastolic murmur or a click.

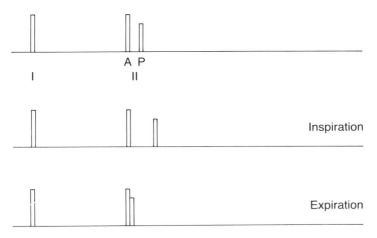

Figure 3.4A Heart sounds
I = 1st heart sound: closure of mitral and tricuspid valves
II = 2nd heart sound: A = aortic valve closure
                       P = pulmonary valve closure
    Pulmonary valve closure is delayed in inspiration and so II appears split: in expiration A
    and P closure are synchronous giving a single 2nd sound.
III = 3rd heart sound is sometimes heard and is due to ventricular filling

---

CAMEO

Sharon Davis is 3. Her doctor saw her at home with a feverish illness. He listened to her chest and heard a loud systolic murmur. He referred her to the paediatrician as an outpatient, but when she attended the clinic there was no murmur.

    She was seen a year later for a routine, pre-school medical and no murmur was heard.

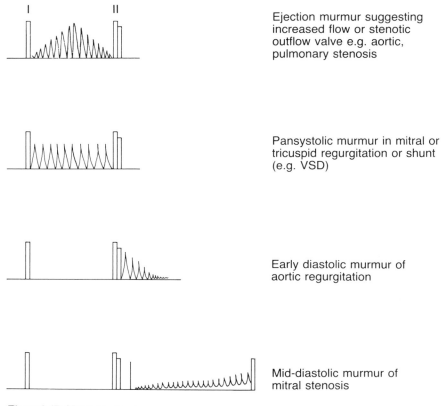

Ejection murmur suggesting increased flow or stenotic outflow valve e.g. aortic, pulmonary stenosis

Pansystolic murmur in mitral or tricuspid regurgitation or shunt (e.g. VSD)

Early diastolic murmur of aortic regurgitation

Mid-diastolic murmur of mitral stenosis

Figure 3.4B Heart murmurs

3.5
Electrocardiology

The electrocardiogram (ECG) is an investigative tool which makes use of the fact that electrical activity, occurring in the heart, can be recorded from the surface of the body in a simple and non-invasive way.

WHO CAN USE IT?

Any doctor can gain useful information from an ECG. The extent to which he uses it and the amount of information he gains from it will depend on his level of knowledge and on his enthusiasm.

It is possible to memorise, or carry, a list of simple, basic rules which enable anyone to extract a small, though useful, amount of information from an ECG tracing with a minimum amount of knowledge or real understanding. This is better than nothing, but, if the rules can be related to what is actually happening in the heart, the tool can become a much more powerful source of information.

Electrocardiology can be a complex and difficult subject, the source of endless controversy amongst the most erudite experts. It is, therefore, not surprising that many GPs hesitate to make as much use as they might of what, at its most basic level, is little more complicated than taking and interpreting the blood pressure.

Individual doctors can develop whatever level of expertise they choose. What is important, as in all areas of medical practice, is for each to know his own limitations: to recognise when he needs help or advice from someone more expert than himself.

HOW SHOULD IT BE USED?

Some important precautions are necessary in the recording and interpretation of an ECG tracing. This chapter aims to describe these, the main elements of the normal ECG and some of the commoner abnormalities which are likely to be encountered in general practice. It should be used in conjunction with the section on electrophysiology (Chapter 1.4 p.31).

We make suggestions about what problems might best be referred and recommend some books which anyone interested in studying the subject further might find useful. We have included a small amount of basic theory.

ECG findings are also referred to, throughout the book, under the headings of individual diseases.

The main points needed for the recognition of a normal ECG are summarised at the end of this chapter. They can be copied and carried about for quick reference. The more often they are used, the less often they will be needed.

When is an ECG useful?

(1)　For the reassurance of the nervous patient or doctor.

(2)　In routine medical examinations and as a baseline for the future.

(3)　In the identification and differentiation of arrhythmias.

(4)　As a diagnostic aid in patients with symptoms or signs suggestive of heart disease.

(5)　In the assessment of hypertension.

(6)　In long-term monitoring of the progress of cardiovascular disease.

What are its limitations?

A normal record does not signify freedom from heart disease: it is usual in early ischaemic heart disease and it does not exclude severe heart disease or early myocardial infarction. Interpretation can be difficult.

HOW DOES IT WORK?

The ECG machine records electrical activity on squared paper, moving at 25 mm per second.

This means that each large square represents 0.2 sec, and each small square 0.04 sec, along the length of the paper.

In the vertical dimension, the machine is usually calibrated so that a voltage of 1 millivolt produces an excursion from the base line of 10 mm (see Figure 3.5A).

All activity in the heart is associated with the passage of electrical current (see section on electrophysiology in Chapter 1.4). This is recorded, in the ECG, by leads attached to the surface of the body.

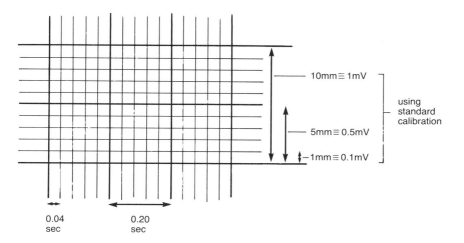

Figure 3.5A ECG paper with measurements
Waves 1 large square (0.2 sec) apart are occurring at a rate of 300/min
Waves 2 large squares (0.4 sec) apart are occurring at a rate of 150/min
Waves 3 large squares (0.6 sec) apart are occurring at a rate of 100/min
Waves 4 large squares (0.8 sec) apart are occurring at a rate of 75/min
15 large squares = 3 sec
No. of beats in 15 large squares x 20 = rate/minute

Current flowing:
towards an electrode is recorded as a positive deflection ;
away from an electrode is recorded as negative;
at right angles to an electrode causes no deflection.

Figure 3.5B shows what would be the appearance if a recording were taken from a single strip of muscle during depolarisation.

The heart consists of two pairs of muscular chambers which contract in sequence.

Current flows through the heart in different directions in relation to each electrode. The resulting tracing (Figure 3.5C) is the basic ECG wave form.

- The P wave represents atrial depolarisation;

- The P – R interval is isoelectric (on the base line) and corresponds to the time taken for the excitation wave to reach the left ventricle via the A – V node;

- The QRS complex is due to ventricular depolarisation. It is the largest deflection because it represents the largest muscle mass:

115

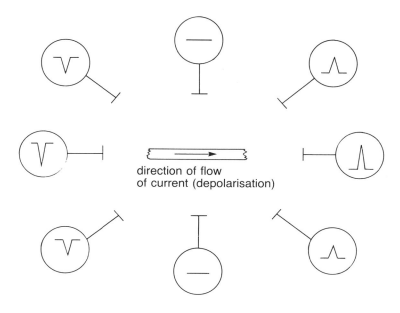

direction of flow
of current (depolarisation)

Figure 3.5B A single strip vector

- the Q wave is the first downward deflection after the P–R interval;
- the R wave is the first upward deflection;
- the S wave is the negative deflection which follows an R wave.

- The T wave is the result of ventricular repolarisation.

The terms:
Depolarisation leads to contraction of cardiac muscle fibres, i.e. systole.

Repolarisation has to occur before the muscle can contract again. This is during diastole.

The base line is the level of electrical activity between contractions.

The voltage (height or depth of deflection) is proportional to the size of the muscle mass, the electrical activity of which it is recording.

When referring to Q, R and S waves, it is conventional to use capital letters to denote large deflections and lower case letters to denote small deflections.

116

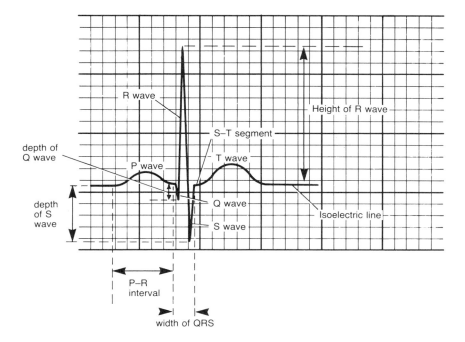

Figure 3.5C The basic tracing, with P, QRS, and T waves; P – R interval and baseline
P – R interval: 0.12 – 0.22 sec
QRS duration: not more than 0.10 sec
q waves: not more than 0.04 sec
　　　　　 not more than ¼ height of ensuing R wave
S in V1 + R in V6: not more than 40 mm
S – T segment should be not more than 1 mm above or below the isoelectric line

THE LEADS

The way the limb leads are attached is a matter of tradition and causes much confusion. It is simpler to consider the chest, or precordial, leads first.

The chest leads

QRS shape

V1: – the positive deflection (R wave) is produced by the right ventricle;
　　　 – the negative deflection (S wave) is produced by the left ventricle;
　　　 – since the mass of the left ventricle is greater than the right, the QRS complex is predominantly negative

117

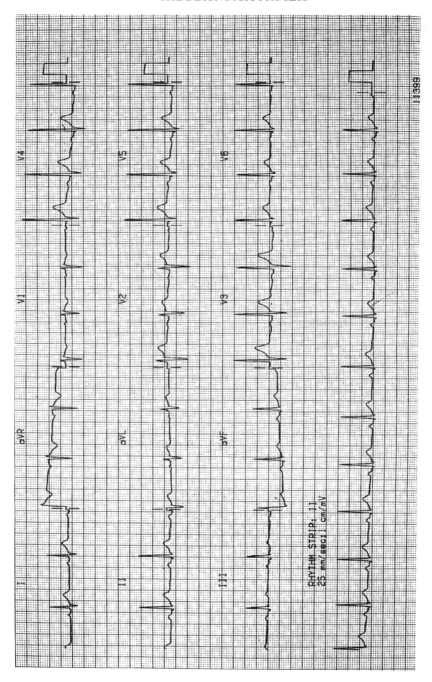

RHYTHM STRIP: II
25 mm/sec; 1 cm/mV

Figure 3.5D Normal ECG

- the complex should be rS, i.e. the S wave is larger than the r wave (see Figure 3.5D, lead V1);
- an R wave (as opposed to an r wave) in V1 is abnormal.

V6:
- the R wave is produced by the left ventricle;
- the s wave is produced by the right ventricle;
- the complex is predominantly positive;
- the R wave is taller than the s wave is deep;
- the appearance is: qR, R, Rs or qRs.

V1 – 6:
- the R wave should increase in size in a progressive manner between these leads, although, in V5 and 6, it may begin to diminish. Thus R V4 should be bigger than R V3 and so on (see Figure 3.5D, V1 – 6).
- the point at which the R and S waves are of equal size is called the transition point (Figure 3.5D, V1 – 6: the transition point is between V2 and V3). The earlier this occurs in the sequence (V1 – 6), the more the left ventricle is predominating.
- This depends on:
  - the position of the heart in the body;
  - the relative mass of the two ventricles.

QRS dimensions

(1) The time from the beginning of the q wave to the end of the S wave should be not more than than 0.10 sec (2.5 small squares).

(2) R waves: at least one should be more than 8 mm high, the tallest should be not more than 27 mm.

(3) S + R: the S wave in V1 and the R wave in V6 should add up to not more than 40 mm.

(4) q waves should be less than a quarter of the height of the R wave which follows and not more than 0.04 sec (one small square) duration.

P – R interval

The interval should be not greater than 0.2 sec (one large square).

T waves

- In V1: the T waves may be upright, flat or inverted.

– In V2: T waves are usually upright. They may be flat or inverted if they were so in V1.

– In V3–6 (Figure 3.5D): T waves are always upright.

S – T segments

These should be not more than 1 mm above the isoelectric line (Figure 3.5D, p.118) and smoothly curved, not flat.

THE LIMB LEADS

The limb leads are: I, II, III, aVR, aVL and aVF.

It helps if these are thought of as if they were attached to the corners of an equilateral triangle with the apex pointing downwards (Figure 3.5E).

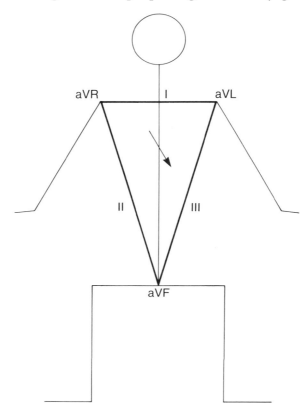

Figure 3.5E The body with triangle superimposed

Leads aVR, aVL and aVF

The augmented limb leads, aVR, aVL and aVF, are unipolar. This means that they record electrical activity in the heart from different directions in a similar way to the precordial leads.

aVR: aVR, recording from the upper right apex of the triangle (the right shoulder), is pointing into the cavity of the heart. (Leads which do this are sometimes called cavity leads.) Most of the electrical current is flowing away from aVR and so the tracing is predominantly, negative including the P waves.

aVL: this can be thought of as recording from the left shoulder.

aVF: this can be thought of as recording from the pubic symphysis.

Leads I, II and III

Unlike the precordial and augmented limb leads, these are bipolar leads. This leads to some very complex theory. However, use can be made of the tracings they produce without understanding it.

The limb leads give an overall view of the heart, contrasting with the close-up produced by the precordial leads. This is because they are all recording from a distance.

P waves

These are:
- best seen in lead II;
- should be smooth and rounded;
- not more than 2.5 mm tall;
- not longer than 0.12 sec (three small squares).

QRS complexes

See p.122 for the electrical axis of the heart.

(1)   The q waves can be ignored:
- in aVR and III always;
- in aVF if the heart is vertical;
- in aVL if the heart is horizontal
  (when these, in effect, become cavity leads: see above).

121

(2)   The q waves in I, II, aVL and aVF (other than in the above circum-
       stances) should be:
       − not more than a quarter of the height of the R wave which follows;
       − not more than 0.01 sec (one small square) in duration (Figure 3.5D
       [p.118], leads I, II, III, aVR, aVL, aVF).

       These are the same criteria as used in the chest leads.

(3)   The R waves:
       − in aVL should be less than 13 mm high;
       − in aVF should be less than 20 mm high (see Figure 3.5D, p.118).

S − T segments (Figure 3.5D, p.118)

These should:
       − be within 1 mm of the isoelectric line;
       − be smoothly rounded or curve gently upwards (not flat);
       − not be trusted in lead III where they can be ignored.

T waves

The T waves should be in the same direction as the QRS complexes in the
same lead. Therefore, if the qRS is predominantly positive (upright), the T
wave should also be positive.

What is the electrical axis of the heart?

The electrical axis is the sum of all the electrical vectors (Figure 3.5F). It is
important because it affects the interpretation of the ECG and also because
it is altered by certain disease processes.

How is the electrical axis measured?

Accurate measurement is unnecessary. As a rough guide:
       − if leads I and II (Figure 3.5G) are both positive, the axis is normal;
       − if lead I is negative (Figure 3.5H), this suggests right axis deviation;
       − if lead II is negative (Figure 3.5I), this suggests left axis deviation.
In the absence of disease, the direction of the axis depends on the patient's
build: tall, thin people tend to have vertical hearts (RAD); short, broad
people tend to have horizontal hearts (LAD). An abnormal axis can be

obscured by the patient's build. Therefore, diagnostic conclusions should not be drawn from the electrical axis alone.

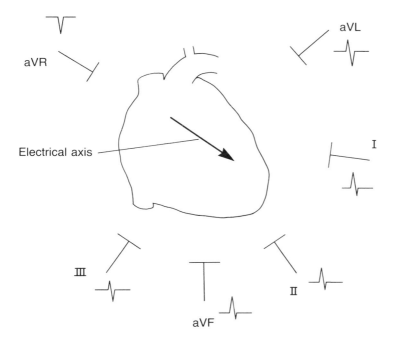

Figure 3.5F Diagram of vectors
In aVR, the current (electrical axis) is flowing away from the electrode and the deflection is therefore negative.
In I and II, the current is flowing towards the electrodes and the deflection is predominantly positive

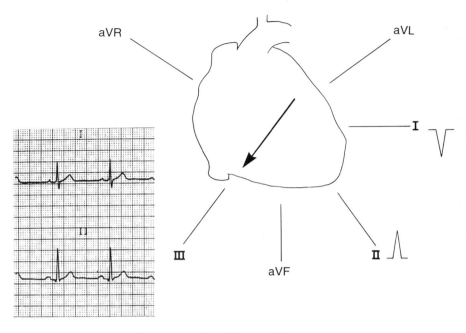

Figure 3.5G Normal electrical axis: leads I and II are positive

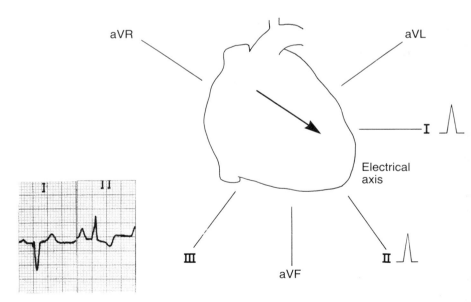

Figure 3.5H Right axis deviation: lead I negative, lead II positive

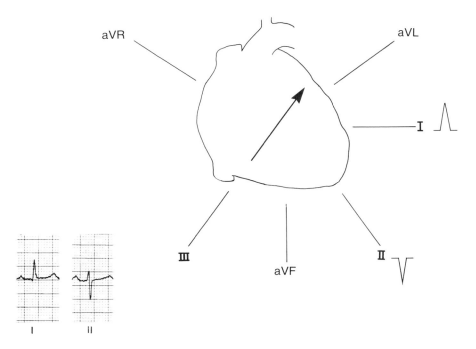

Figure 3.5I Left axis deviation: lead I positive, lead II negative

WHAT CAN THE ECG TELL YOU?

The ECG is never used in isolation in the confirmation of health or in the diagnosis of disease. It provides additional information which is used together with all the other clinical findings in the elucidation of a clinical problem. Sometimes it adds little to what is already known; at others it provides the answer to a puzzle. (See also Chapter 1.4 on Electrophysiology and Chapter 4.5 on Arrhythmias.)

A normal ECG does not tell you that the patient has a normal heart.

A truly abnormal ECG is not compatible with health but the range of normality is wide and it may be unwise to label anyone as having heart disease on the basis of an abnormal ECG alone.

Factors to consider

Rhythm and rate: the timing and sequence of the electrical events in the heart

– can be seen in any lead but leads II or V1 are most often used because P

125

waves are most clearly seen in these leads: a rhythm strip of at least 10 beats is useful.

- rate ranges from 60 to 100 per min. There are two quick methods of calculating it:
    - count the number of large squares between R waves and divide into 300:
        2 large squares = rate of 150/min
        3 large squares = rate of 100/min
        4 large squares = rate of 75/min
        5 large squares = rate of 60/min
        6 large squares = rate of 50/min.
    - count the number of small squares between R waves and divide into 1500.
    - if the rhythm is irregular, count the number of complexes in 30 large squares (6 sec) and multiply by 10.
    - P waves must:
        - be regular;
        - be uniform in each lead;
        - have a regular one-to-one relationship with the QRS complexes.
    - P – R interval must be:
        - between 0.12 sec (3 small squares) and 0.20 sec (one large or five small squares).

Conduction

This is reflected in many aspects of the recording:
- electrical axis
- P – R interval
- width of QRS complexes
- constant one-to-one relationship between P waves and QRS complexes.

Condition of the myocardium

The following indicators are well seen in the chest leads:
- voltages;
- S – T segments;
- T waves;
- R wave progression.

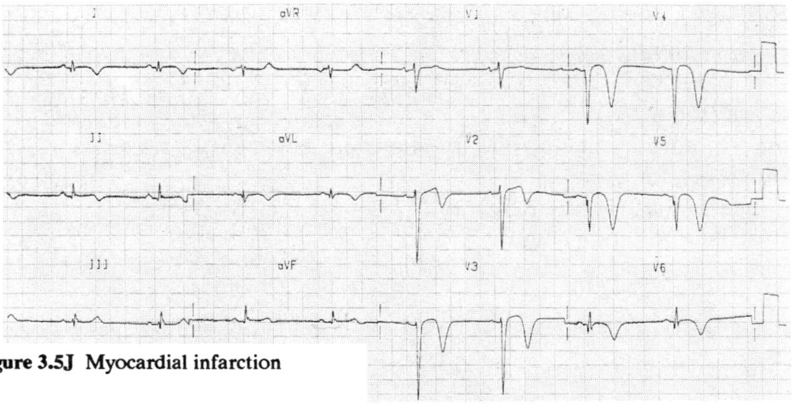

Figure 3.5J Myocardial infarction

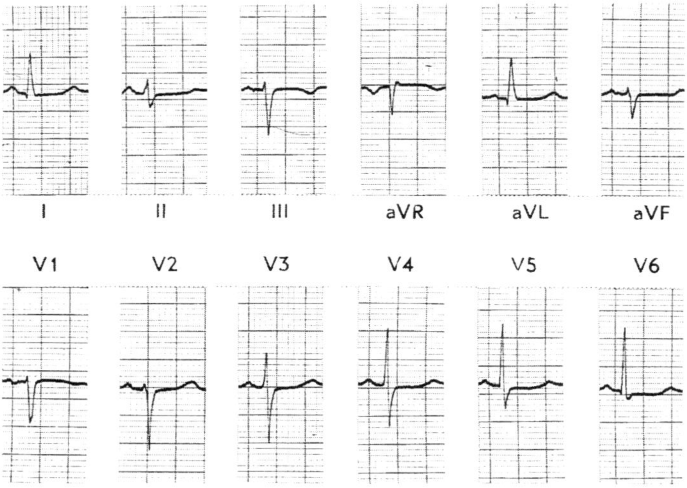

Figure 3.5K Ischaemia

What abnormalities may the ECG show?

Signs of myocardial damage

These are (see p.179):
- pathological q waves;
- S – T elevation or depression of more than 1 mm;
- T wave inversion;
- loss of normal R wave progression;
     (all of which occur in myocardial infarction (Figure 3.5J).
- Flat S – T segments and T waves which occur in ischaemia (Figure 3.5K).

127

Signs of arrhythmia

These are (see p.238):
- loss of normal one-to-one relationship between P waves and QRS complexes, for example:
    - heart block (Figure 3.5L);
    - atrial fibrillation (Figure 3.5M).

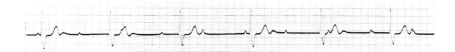

Figure 3.5L Heart block

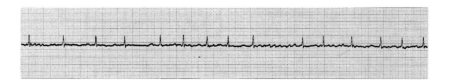

Figure 3.5M Atrial fibrillation

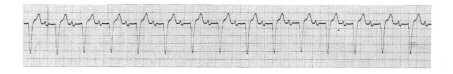

Figure 3.5N First degree heart block

- Abnormalities of P–R interval, for example:
    - long in first degree heart block (Figure 3.5N);
    - short in ventricular pre-excitation* (Figure 3.5O).
- Increased width of QRS complexes (if in sinus rhythm), for example:
    - right bundle branch block (RSR´ pattern in V1) (Figure 3.5P);
    - left bundle branch block (no RSR´ pattern)* (Figure 3.5Q).

---

* These two are of particular importance when it comes to interpreting the ECG. Normal criteria cannot be applied if ventricular pre-excitation or left bundle branch block are present.

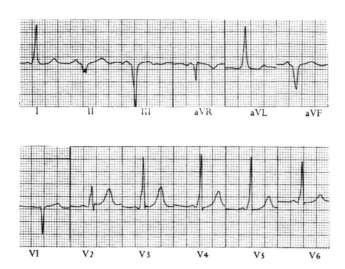

Figure 3.5O Wolff – Parkinson – White syndrome (ventricular pre-excitation)

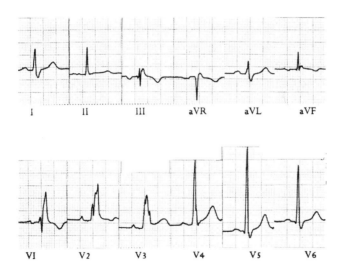

Figure 3.5P Right bundle branch block

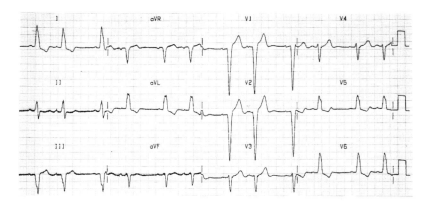

Figure 3.5Q Left bundle branch block

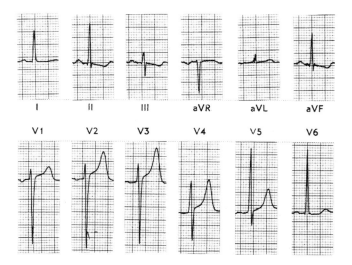

Figure 3.5R Left ventricular hypertrophy

Signs of muscle hypertrophy

- S in V1 + R in V6 greater than normal, for example:
  - left ventricular hypertrophy (Figure 3.5R);
  - (left ventricular hypertrophy does not cause left axis deviation).

- right axis deviation, for example:
  - right ventricular hypertrophy (Figure 3.5S).

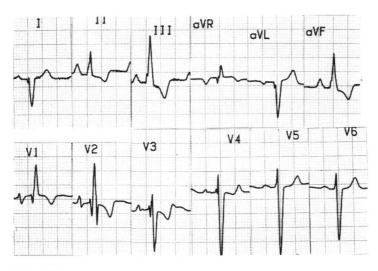

Figure 3.5S RAD

RULES FOR INTERPRETATION OF AN ECG

(1) Check: name, date, calibration;
              quality of recording: interference, baseline drift.

(2) Is there sinus rhythm (P wave before every qRS)?

(3) Is the P – R interval less than 0.12 sec (three small squares)?
If it is, then pre-excitation may be present and render interpretation of the rest of the ECG difficult.

(4) Is there LBBB (wide qRS; no RSR´ in V1)?
If so, qRS, S – T segments and T waves will be abnormal and cannot be used as indicators of disease.

Assuming no pre-excitation and no LBBB, look at:

(5) Precordial leads:
- QRS shape: V1: rS
             V6: qR (or R, qRs or Rs)
             V1 – 6: normal R wave progression.
- QRS measurements:
  - (i)   duration: 0.10 sec (2.5 small squares)
  - (ii)   at least one R wave > 8 mm high
  - (iii)   no R taller than 27 mm
  - (iv)   no S deeper than 30 mm
  - (v)   S V1 + R V6 < 40 mm
  - (vi)   q < one quarter the height of following R.
- T waves:
V1: variable but should be similar to previous recordings
V2: upright (usually)
V3 – 6: upright.
- S – T segments: < 1mm away from isoelectric line.

(6) Limb leads:
- q waves: – normal in aVR and III
               – < one quarter the height of following R in other leads
- R waves: in aVL: 13 – 20 mm
- Electrical axis. Leads I and II should be positive
- T waves: same direction as qRS in same lead
- S – T segments: as for precordial leads.

POINTS

- a normal ECG does not exclude heart disease
- an unusual looking tracing may be normal for that patient
- if really puzzled, take another recording, reapplying and checking the attachment of the leads
- if patient's condition good but ECG doubtful, repeat next day
- write a report on each ECG

WHO SHOULD BE REFERRED?

Any doubtful ECG should be sent to a cardiologist for interpretation. He or she is likely to want to see the patient as well.

The following points may help:

(1)   The range of normal is so great that it sometimes requires an expert to decide whether an apparently abnormal ECG in fact indicates disease at all.

(2)   The criteria given in this chapter should be used as guidelines only. There will be exceptions to them.

(3)   Arrhythmias are particularly difficult to sort out and accurate diagnosis is needed for management (see Chapter 4.5 p.238).

(4)   Non-specific S – T changes are common and difficult to interpret.

HOW TO MAKE AN ECG RECORDING
(to be pasted inside lid of machine)

1. The patient should be lying comfortably, as warm and as relaxed as possible.
2. Switch on machine to warm up.
3. Attach limb leads, according to markings, using electrode jelly.
4. Run for a short time on 'test' to check for interference and baseline drift.
5. Check calibration: 1 mV = 2 large squares.
6. Write patient's name and date at beginning of strip.
7. Check leads are attached correctly.
8. Record leads I, II, III, aVR, aVL, aVF in that order:
    three beats in each lead unless otherwise indicated.
9. Apply and record chest leads, V1–6 in turn, as shown in diagram below. Make sure jelly does not spread between recording points.
10. Record rhythm strip, lead II, 8–10 beats.
11. Label leads on tracing.
12. Remove leads, checking that they were correctly attached.
13. Wash and dry electrodes and straps.

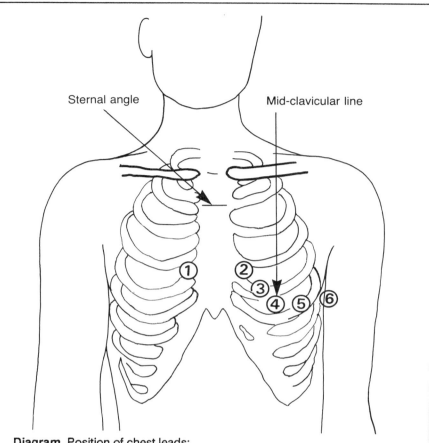

Diagram Position of chest leads:
1. Junction of 4th right intercostal space and sternal border
2. Junction of 4th left intercostal space and sternal border
3. Mid-way between points 2 and 4
4. 5th intercostal space in the midclavicular line
5. Left anterior axillary line horizontally from 4
6. Left mid-axillary line at the same horizontal level as 4 and 5

3.6
Pathological Tests and Chest X-rays

Most GPs now have access to a laboratory for pathological investigations but they have to be used economically and selectively and with a clear objective. Pathological investigations may be needed:

(1)   As part of the diagnostic process
(2)   To monitor treatment
(3)   To monitor progress of disease
(4)   For screening.

HAEMATOLOGY TESTS

Haemoglobin
- To exclude anaemia in patients with recent onset of:
  - angina
  - intermittent claudication
  - heart failure;

- In suspected sub-acute bacterial endocarditis (SBE).

White blood cell count (WBC)
- In suspected infections such as SBE, pericarditis.

Erythrocyte sedimentation rate (ESR)
- Raised in SBE (usually), inflammatory conditions, rheumatic fever.

BIOCHEMICAL TESTS

Blood urea and electrolytes
These should be measured
- in hypertension:
  - low potassium in Conn's syndrome
  - high sodium in Cushing's syndrome
  - urea and creatinine raised when renal function impaired.
- in arrhythmias:
  - serum potassium level.

- in heart failure:
  - as an initial baseline
  - to monitor effects of treatment.
- before starting certain drugs and during treatment:
  - digoxin
  - diuretics
  - ACE inhibitors.

Blood sugar is used in the diagnosis and monitoring of diabetes.

Liver function tests are used in monitoring patients on certain drugs, for example amiodarone.

Cardiac enzymes are used to confirm diagnosis of acute myocardial infarction (see p.189).

Thyroid function tests are used to:
- Diagnose thyroid dysfunction, e.g. recent onset of:
  - arrhythmias
  - angina
  - heart failure.
- Monitor patients taking amiodarone.

Lipoproteins
- Screening of patients at risk of ischaemic heart disease (IHD).
- Monitoring of patients with hyperlipidaemia.

Prothrombin time is used before and during treatment with warfarin.

Fibrinogen levels
This test is not widely used at present but fibrinogen is known to be a factor in the pathogenesis of myocardial infarction and it may be used in the future.

Urine
- Albumen to detect renal damage:
  - nephritis
  - nephrotic syndrome
  - hypertension.
- Glucose: diabetes?
- Microscopy:
  - red cells (SBE)
  - casts (acute nephritis).
- Culture: infection.

CHEST X-RAYS

Most GPs have access to chest X-rays but do not have the opportunity of seeing the films themselves. It is a great advantage to see the films for yourself and to develop some facility in understanding them.

When do you need a chest X-ray?

As part of the diagnostic process

(1)   In a patient who is breathless, to help differentiate between left heart failure and other causes. If LHF is present when the film is taken, there will be evidence of it.

(2)   In angina: to check for evidence of cardiomyopathy or valve disease.

(3)   To help in diagnosis, when a murmur has been picked up on routine examination.

For monitoring

(1)   To monitor treatment, especially of heart failure.

(2)   To monitor progress of the disease, for instance, the size of the heart in a patient with a cardiomyopathy; the size of the left atrium in someone with mitral valve disease.

What do you look for?

Heart shadow
Great vessels
Vasculature and fluid in the lung fields
Rib notching.

Heart shadow

- Overall size is never normally greater than 16 cm on a standard film.

- May be impossible to distinguish cardiomegaly from pericardial effusion.

- *Cardio-thoracic ratio*: this is the ratio of the size of the heart compared with the size of the chest. As a rough guide, it should be not more than 50% but varies according to stature and build. It is usually expressed in cm as a fraction, e.g. 14.5/30 (or 145/300 mm). Comparison of heart size on successive films is useful in monitoring progress.

- *Chamber enlargement*: it is sometimes possible to diagnose the enlargement of one or more chambers, particularly if they are dilated, e.g. left ventricle in aortic regurgitation, left atrium in mitral stenosis.

Great vessels

- Aorta:
    - calcification in the aortic valve can be seen best on a lateral film;
    - dilated in: elderly, aortic stenosis, aortic aneurysm.

- Pulmonary artery:
    - dilated in: pulmonary stenosis, L R shunts.

Lung fields

(1)   Vasculature:
    - upper lobe veins dilated in pulmonary venous congestion. They are not normally more than 3 mm in diameter on a standard film;
    - all veins congested in pulmonary oedema;
    - arteries over-filled in L-to-R shunts;
    - arteries under-filled in pulmonary stenosis;

(2)   Fluid:
    - interstitial/interlobar/pleural in left heart failure;
    - hilar flare (bat-wing appearance) in acute LHF.

Rib notching

This is seen in coarctation of the aorta.

PART 4:
CARDIAC DISEASE

4.1
Introduction

In this part of *Commonsense Cardiology* specific diseases and clinico-pathological states are described in detail:

In parallel with Chapter 2.3 on Sorting Out the Drugs and Chapter 3.3 on Sorting Out the Symptoms, the chapters in this part, particularly those concerned with pathological conditions, are all set out to a similar pattern. This takes the form of describing the condition by answering commonsense questions such as what is it, who gets it, what are its causes and effects? How can it be prevented? What are the symptoms? What else could it be? What investigations should be carried out? How is it treated and what are the likely outcomes?

Whenever it is appropriate, detailed guidelines are provided for management of the patient, including discussion of the relative advantages of home care and hospital admission.

Underlying causes or different ways in which a condition manifests itself may be treated separately (but in the same manner) as subsections within particular chapters. For instance, included in Ischaemic Heart Disease are separate sections on angina and myocardial infarction which almost constitute chapters in themselves.

4.2
Ischaemic Heart Disease

INTRODUCTION

Ischaemic heart disease (IHD) is a local manifestation of a generalised disease process: atheroma. It may occur in apparent isolation, affecting only the coronary arteries with little disease elsewhere, or as part of extensive disease throughout the arterial system.

This chapter begins with a discussion of atheroma, its general causes, effects and prevention before relating this specifically to ischaemic heart disease.

Ischaemic heart disease (IHD) is not a uniform process affecting everyone in the same way. It can present a great variety of symptoms and signs, depending on which of the coronary arteries are most affected and whether the disease affects mostly peripheral or proximal vessels. The reason for individual variation in the way the disease behaves is obscure. Its manifestations can be broadly divided into five groups:

4.2.1   Sudden cardiac death
4.2.2   Silent ischaemia
4.2.3   Ischaemic cardiomyopathy
4.2.4   Angina
4.2.5   Myocardial infarction.

There is considerable overlap between the last four: many people show signs of all four, others of only one, but there are differences between them. In the sections which follow, they will be considered separately, whilst acknowledging that they often coexist.

Ischaemic heart disease is also a common cause of heart failure and of arrhythmias (see Chapters 4.3 and 4.5).

ATHEROMA

What is atheroma?

Atheroma is the deposition of fatty substances in the walls of large and medium-sized arteries.

A crack appears in the endothelium lining an artery and is sealed with platelets and fibrin. Later, cholesterol is taken up by the fibrin and a plaque of atheroma forms. The endothelium may grow over the plaque. If it does not, then a roughened surface is left, causing more platelets to accumulate and enlarge the plaque (Figure 4.2A). There is also a proliferation of fibroblasts as part of the healing process.

These factors facilitate the process:
– hyperlipidaemia
– hypertension
– smoking.

What is hyperlipidaemia?

Fats are carried in the blood as cholesterol and triglycerides. Cholesterol is used in the body for the synthesis of cell membranes, hormones and bile acids. Most of the cholesterol comes from the diet, although synthesis can occur in the liver and small intestine. It is insoluble in water and so is transported combined with protein in the form of lipoprotein.

The lipoproteins can be separated into various fractions according to their molecular weight:

(1) Low-density lipoproteins (LDL) supply cholesterol to the peripheral tissues. If present in excess, they are deposited in the arterial walls and contribute to the formation of atheroma. Thus, a high level of LDL in the serum is associated with a high risk of ischaemic heart disease.

(2) High-density lipoproteins (HDL) contain esterified cholesterol, which has been removed from the peripheral tissues and is on the way back to the liver to be excreted in the bile. A high proportion of HDL is associated with a low risk of ischaemic heart disease.

(3) Total cholesterol (TC): the biochemical results are usually expressed as a ratio of cholesterol to HDL. The laboratory measures total cholesterol (TC) and LDL. HDL is then found by subtraction:

$$HDL = TC - LDL$$

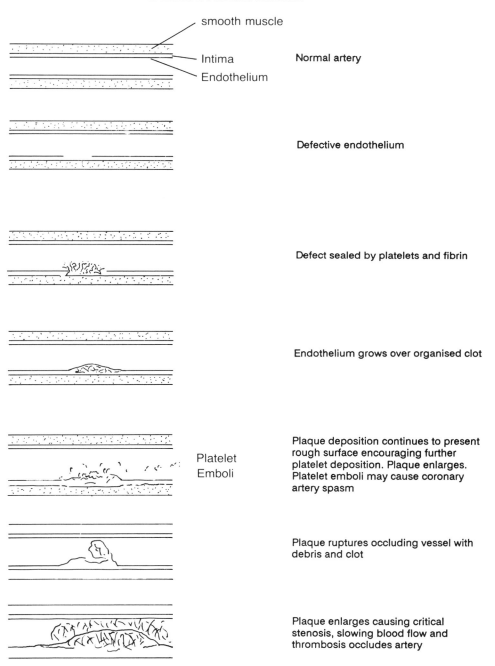

smooth muscle

Intima

Endothelium

Normal artery

Defective endothelium

Defect sealed by platelets and fibrin

Endothelium grows over organised clot

Platelet Emboli

Plaque deposition continues to present rough surface encouraging further platelet deposition. Plaque enlarges. Platelet emboli may cause coronary artery spasm

Plaque ruptures occluding vessel with debris and clot

Plaque enlarges causing critical stenosis, slowing blood flow and thrombosis occludes artery

Figure 4.2A Atheromatous plaque formation

The normal range is $1-1.5$ mmol/l. High figures carry reduced risk for IHD.

When calculating the risk, the cholesterol/HDL ratio is used by most laboratories so that the total cholesterol is included:

$$Ratio = TC/HDL$$

The normal range is 3 to 6. Higher figures carry an increased risk of IHD.

Triglycerides are also derived from dietary fat but they can be synthesised in the liver from carbohydrates and free fatty acids. These are transported to peripheral tissues by very-low-density lipoproteins (VLDL) in response to high carbohydrate and alcohol intake. They are not directly related to high risk of IHD but influence blood clotting factors. The triglycerides are broken down in muscle and adipose tissue to glycerol and free fatty acids. These are used for energy and storage. Dietary triglycerides are carried in chylomicrons, which give the serum a turbid appearance after a fatty meal.

Table 4.2A Types of lipoprotein

Lipoprotein	Characteristics
LDL	Rich in cholesterol High level associated with high risk of IHD Lowering level can reduce risk of IHD
HDL	Contains esterified cholesterol [safe] High level associated with low risk of IHD
VLDL	Rich in triglycerides

Why does hyperlipidaemia matter?

There is a direct relationship between the level of serum cholesterol and the incidence of IHD (Figure 4.2B).

Who has hyperlipidaemia?

Hereditary hyperlipidaemia

A small number of people have a genetic predisposition to hyperlipidaemia. Some of these have familial hypercholesterolaemia (FH). This affects about

1 in 500 of the population so that, on average, every GP might be expected to have four or five patients with this condition. In fact, since it runs in families, it is very uneven and some doctors have considerably more than this. Screening is discussed in Chapter 5.3.

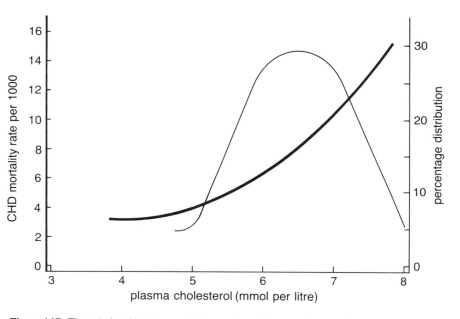

Figure 4.2B The relationship between ischaemic heart disease and serum cholesterol

Dietary hyperlipidaemia

The main cause of hyperlipidaemia is dietary. In countries, such as Africa, where diets are low in animal fat, the average serum cholesterol is about 4.5 mmol/l and IHD is rare.

In Britain, 64% of people aged between 25 and 59 have a cholesterol level of over 5.2 mmol/l – a significant risk of IHD – and 23% over 6.5 mmol/l – a high risk of IHD.

The majority of the population in Britain have serum cholesterol levels which put them at significant risk of IHD and this is borne out by the high incidence and mortality rate of the disease in this country.

Primary prevention is discussed in Chapter 5.3.

Secondary prevention

Figure 4.2C shows a protocol for the organisation of screening for hyperlipidaemia. In patients found to have raised serum cholesterol, the possibility of secondary hyperlipidaemia due to an underlying cause should be considered.

Table 4.2B Secondary hyperlipidaemia

	Cholesterol	Triglyceride
Diabetes mellitus	–	+ +
Hypothyroidism	+ +	–
Nephrotic syndrome	+ +	+
Uraemia	–	+
Primary biliary cirrhosis	+ +	–
Alcoholism	–	+
Oral contraceptives	–	+
Beta-blockers	–	+
Thiazide diuretics	+	–

Treatment

General advice should be given to everyone to reduce animal fat in the diet, including dairy products such as eggs, butter, milk and cheese, to eat fish especially oily fish, poultry and lentils instead of red meat, to substitute soft margarine, powdered or skimmed milk and cook with vegetable oils, to increase the content of fibre in the diet by eating wholemeal bread and adding bran, especially oat bran, and to reduce the content of unrefined carbohydrate by avoiding sugar, sweets and puddings and also alcohol. This is particularly important in patients with high triglycerides.

If the serum cholesterol does not fall below 7.5 mmol/l following a careful diet, a serious risk of IHD exists and treatment with drugs is indicated.

(1) Cholestyramine causes triglycerides to rise so is most useful if the triglycerides are low and the LDL cholesterol high (>5 mmol/l). Individual patients may need from 12 to 36 g daily but few patients can cope with the full dosage regime. The early morning dose is the most important so they should be encouraged to take this even if they default on those later in the day. The drug is easier to tolerate if instructions for taking it are carefully followed:

ISCHAEMIC HEART DISEASE

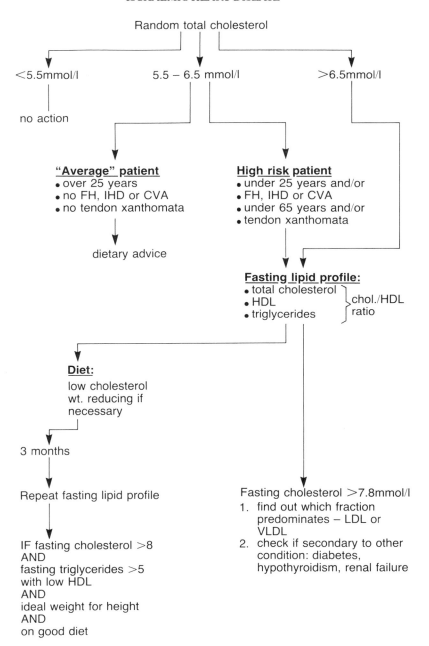

Random total cholesterol

<5.5mmol/l   5.5 – 6.5 mmol/l   >6.5mmol/l

no action

"Average" patient
- over 25 years
- no FH, IHD or CVA
- no tendon xanthomata

dietary advice

High risk patient
- under 25 years and/or
- FH, IHD or CVA
- under 65 years and/or
- tendon xanthomata

Fasting lipid profile:
- total cholesterol
- HDL   } chol./HDL
- triglycerides } ratio

Diet:
low cholesterol
wt. reducing if
necessary

3 months

Repeat fasting lipid profile

IF fasting cholesterol >8
AND
fasting triglycerides >5
with low HDL
AND
ideal weight for height
AND
on good diet

Fasting cholesterol >7.8mmol/l
1. find out which fraction
   predominates – LDL or
   VLDL
2. check if secondary to other
   condition: diabetes,
   hypothyroidism, renal failure

THEN REFER and/or treat with drugs in addition to diet

Figure 4.2C Protocol for hyperlipidaemia screening

149

(i)   each dose should be mixed with water and washed down with more water.

(ii)   each dose should be followed by food. If the patient is not about to have a meal, the dose should be omitted.

(2)   Fibrates, e.g. gemfibrozil, can be given to all patients with hyper-lipidaemia and are especially useful in those with raised triglyceride levels. The dose is 600 mg twice daily.

(3)   Cholestyramine and gemfibrozil given together make a satisfactory and well-tolerated regime for many patients. The cholestyramine is given as a single dose in the evening.

    The use of lipid-lowering drugs should always be combined with diet. MaxEPA (extracted from oily fish) lowers VLDL but has no effect on LDL cholesterol.

What is the effect of atheroma?

At an early stage, atheroma narrows the affected artery and reduces flow through it. Later, the atheroma may itself totally obstruct the artery or it may slow the flow to such an extent that only a small group of sticky platelets is needed to complete the obstruction.

    The effect of total obstruction of any artery depends on the organ involved and on the extent of collateral circulation which is available to supply the region. This, in turn, depends on the health of neighbouring arteries and on the speed with which the obstruction has formed. If blood flow is reduced gradually over a long period, then numerous collateral arteries may open up, provided they are not themselves starved of blood by diseased proximal arteries.

    It is common for blood flow in atheromatous arteries to be adequate for minimal activity but to be unable to increase when there is increased demand. This accounts for the symptoms of intermittent claudication, abdominal pain after meals (associated with mesenteric atheroma), as well as exertional angina.

    Total loss of blood supply to any tissue results in death of the tissue. Chronic, long-standing ischaemia causes atrophy, fibrosis and loss of function.

    In the heart, the effects of this process vary from one individual to another (see later) but, in all its manifestations, ischaemia of the myocardium causes a loss of contractility. This means that the ability of the heart to increase its output in response to the needs of the body are reduced. This may be very obvious, as in heart failure, or difficult to recognise, as in someone with silent ischaemia or early ischaemic cardiomyopathy.

Ischaemia causes arrhythmias by damaging the conducting system and also by damaging areas of myocardium, which then become irritable and form ectopic foci.

Who gets atheroma?

Anyone may develop atheroma but some people are more at risk than others. These risk factors are discussed at length in Chapter 5.2, p.297. They are:

Smoking
Hyperlipidaemia
Hypertension
Diabetes
Obesity
Alcohol abuse.

The disease is more common, more severe and more extensive in smokers and in diabetics than in other people. It is especially serious in diabetics who smoke. This appears to be due to the way diabetics handle fats. It is essential for diabetics to be non-smokers and it helps if control of their diabetes is as good as it can be. The problem has been made worse by the concentration, until recently, on the low-carbohydrate/free-fat diets which diabetics were advised to follow. Even now, many diabetics have, and adhere to, diets which encourage unlimited eggs and foods containing high levels of saturated fats: sausages, bacon, red meat, butter.

It is particularly important for diabetics to eat healthily. This means a diet low in saturated fats and high in polyunsaturated fats and fish (see Chapter 5.3, p.308).

Hypertension in people with atheroma certainly increases the risks – especially of stroke, myocardial infarction and renal failure.

Peripheral vascular disease almost exclusively affects people who either smoke or have diabetes or both.

The worst outlook is for obese, hypertensive, poorly controlled diabetics, who smoke and have hyperlipidaemia.

What should you do?

It is most important for every doctor to maintain a high index of suspicion for ischaemic heart disease and to recognise that it can present in many different ways. It is the commonest serious disease in the developed world and affects both sexes and all ages. It can show itself with great drama, as sudden death on the squash court, or can be entirely symptomless. The pre-infarction syndrome (see p.164) is a particular challenge to doctors as it provides a potential opportunity for preventing an imminent disaster.

In assessing a patient with ischaemic heart disease, it is important to discover, as far as possible, the extent of atheroma in the rest of the body, especially the brain and legs. This may influence the prognosis and the choice of treatment. For instance, if a patient has obvious peripheral vascular disease, it is better to avoid the use of beta-blockers and it may be inadvisable to carry out heart surgery in a person who has extensive cerebrovascular disease.

4.2.1 SUDDEN CARDIAC DEATH

Sudden cardiac death (SCD) is a common cause of death.

What is it?

Death within an hour of the onset of symptoms.
In about half, the symptoms are virtually instantaneous.

What causes it?

It is usually due to ventricular fibrillation.

At postmortem, coronary artery disease is often extensive but acute myocardial infarction is not usual.

Very few SCDs (less than 5%) occur during strenuous exercise.

In those that do, the exercise is of the anaerobic, 'sprint' type, such as squash, rather than aerobic, 'marathon' type, such as jogging.

Who gets it?

It is especially likely in patients with ventricular dilatation. This means that it is especially common in patients with heart failure.

About 50% of people who die suddenly have previously recognised heart disease but not all have ischaemic heart disease. Heart failure with another underlying cause and aortic stenosis also form part of this group.

Most SCD casualties are male and have a high level of risk factors for IHD,especially hypertension, smoking and diabetes.

What can be done?

Careful treatment of heart failure can reduce the incidence of SCD. Diagnosis and treatment prevents SCD in patients with aortic stenosis and early resuscitation of patients with ventricular fibrillation can save some (Table 4.2C).

Table 4.2C Cardiac resuscitation

1. Note state of consciousness and pupils
2. Feel for carotid pulse
3. Drag patient on to floor (or flat firm surface)
4. Strike one smart blow with fist to lower third of sternum
5. Call for help and send for coronary ambulance
6. Commence external compression lower third of sternum about 60/min
7. Ensure AIRWAY clear by extending neck
8. Block nose and commence mouth to mouth respiration: 2 breaths to every 15 compressions.

When ambulance arrives:
9. Change to airway or endotracheal tube and inflate lungs with bag and oxygen. ECG if available
10. If still no pulse or ECG shows ventricular fibrillation give DC shock – 200 Joules
11. If necessary repeat with 200 Joules, then 400 Joules
12. Transport to hospital as rapidly as possible

4.2.2 SILENT ISCHAEMIA

What is it?

This is a phrase coined recently to describe the condition of people who are found to have ischaemic heart disease, including areas of actual infarction, but who have had no symptoms whatsoever. Patients with angina associated with ECG changes have been shown, by ambulatory monitoring, to have similar changes on occasions when they have no pain. The number of such incidents can be reduced by anti-anginal drugs but it is impossible to tell, clinically, whether they are well controlled or not, because of the absence of symptoms.

The term is sometimes used to include those who suffer myocardial infarction which is painless, but which does produce symptoms of fatigue, arrhythmia or heart failure. It is probably best reserved for the completely symptomless group.

About one quarter of all myocardial infarcts are painless and perhaps half of these are truly silent. An unknown number of people with angina, and some without, have silent ischaemic episodes. It therefore seems that this condition is far more common than was once thought but it is difficult to assess its exact incidence. It is likely that the outlook for people with silent infarction is the same as for other people with the same pathological process so it has to be taken seriously.

What does it do?

It damages the myocardium by causing muscle death in the same way as symptomatic myocardial infarction. This is sometimes found on an ECG taken for some other reason.

It also causes intermittent ischaemia, which is similar to angina except that it is symptomless. This is sometimes found during effort testing, when ECG signs of ischaemia occur without symptoms.

How do you know?

Silent ischaemia can be diagnosed only by ambulatory monitoring.

4.2.3 ISCHAEMIC CARDIOMYOPATHY

What is it?

Atrophy and weakening of the myocardium by chronic ischaemia.

It is usually due to multiple small infarcts, which occur at different times. The remaining myocardial cells hypertrophy and are separated by areas of fibrosis. It is sometimes associated with diffuse fibrosis without actual infarction, so that all the cells survive but each has fewer myofibrils and function is impaired. It is commonly accompanied by angina and its course punctuated by episodes of infarction. The prominent features are heart failure and arrhythmias due to ventricular dilatation and myocardial damage.

What do you do?

Basic preventative measures: i.e. control of smoking, obesity, diet; optimum treatment of associated problems: e.g. angina, heart failure, hypertension; and identification of other factors: e.g. anaemia, thyroid disease, diabetes, renal failure, are all important and can make a significant difference to the outcome.

4.2.4 ANGINA

What is angina?

There have been a number of different definitions but the one we will use is:

Pain due to transient cardiac ischaemia.

Originally, the term angina was used to describe only anterior chest pain radiating into the neck. It is now used by most doctors to mean pain caused by transient cardiac ischaemia, whatever the site of the pain.

Such pain may occur in a number of sites (Figure 4.2D) but is usually consistent for any one individual.

Some patients experience pain in one or more sites, simultaneously.

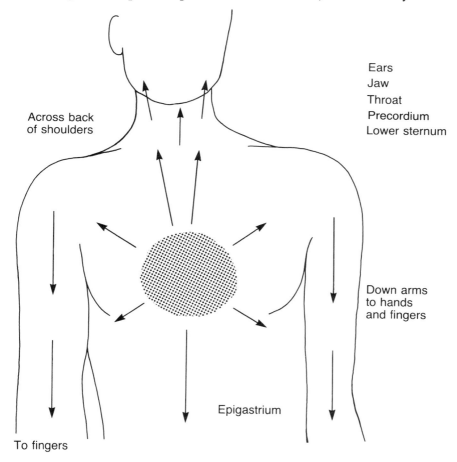

Figure 4.2D Common sites of angina

The commonest type of anginal pain starts retrosternally and radiates across the front of the chest and up into the neck. The less common varieties are frequently not recognised by doctors: patients often fail to mention, or do not observe, any connection with exercise and in fact there may be none (see later). Many teeth have been extracted, tennis elbows injected and gallons of antacids consumed, before the diagnosis has been made.

Angina is a symptom of reduced myocardial perfusion; an indication of coronary atheroma or spasm and not a disease process itself. It may occur alone or together with other symptoms of ischaemic heart disease. The contractility of the myocardium is nearly always reduced, when angina is present, indicating an element of ischaemic cardiomyopathy (see next section).

The reduction in coronary perfusion leads to a reduction in contractility and thence in stroke volume and overall cardiac output. This usually affects the left ventricle to a greater extent than the right and, if heart failure occurs, it is more likely to be left ventricular, at least to start with.

If atrial fibrillation occurs as a complication, the atrial contribution to ventricular filling is lost and stroke volume, and therefore cardiac output, is further reduced. If the atrial fibrillation causes a rapid ventricular rate, ventricular filling is reduced again. Angina may therefore be associated with reduced cardiac output by three mechanisms:

(1)   reduced contractility, due to reduced perfusion and ischaemia;

(2)   reduced ventricular filling, due to loss of atrial contraction;

(3)   reduced ventricular filling, due to reduced filling time, due to increased ventricular rate.

These mechanisms are worth noting because, although all of them reduce cardiac output by reducing stroke volume, the management of each is different. Figure 4.2E shows the relationship between filling and heart rate.

Why does it happen?

Unlike skeletal muscle, myocardial tissue extracts oxygen from blood at a fixed rate. An increased supply of oxygen can only be obtained by an increase in blood flow and not by an increase in the amount extracted. Therefore, the myocardium is especially sensitive to reductions in coronary perfusion due to atheroma.

The mechanism of the pain in angina is not certain but it is associated with a blood flow to the myocardium which is inadequate for its needs at the time. In exertional angina, the pain arises when there is increased demand

156

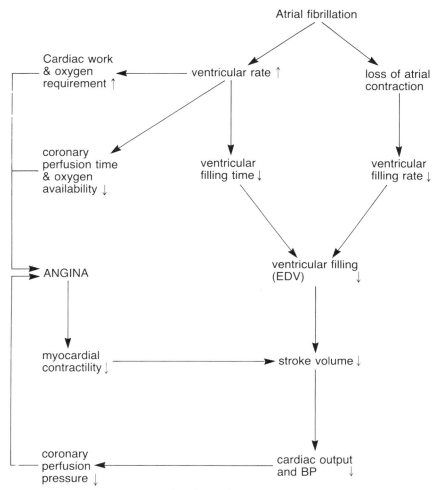

Figure 4.2E Atrial fibrillation precipitating angina

which is not being satisfied, and it goes during rest, when the supply and demand are once again in equilibrium.

In atypical angina, it is not at all clear to what extent spasm of affected arteries is involved, but there is no doubt that this can happen as it has been observed during coronary angiography. It is also not clear whether arteries which cause angina by developing spasm are necessarily diseased or whether spasm can occur in healthy arteries.

Angina is usually associated with atheroma but, in certain circumstances, the atheroma may be minimal and the precipitating cause of the symptom is an increased demand by the myocardium. Anything which makes the heart work harder increases the oxygen needs of the myocardium, and therefore the demand for high coronary perfusion. Even minimal coronary artery disease may make this impossible.

Causes of increased oxygen demand by the myocardium include conditions which increase resistance to LV outflow or raise peripheral resistance (aortic stenosis, hypertension, coarctation); high output states (hyperthyroidism, anaemia) and regurgitant valves.

Tachyarrhythmias precipitate angina by shortening diastole as well as by increasing work. Diastole is the time during which coronary perfusion takes place and perfusion is reduced by any increase in heart rate.

What is it like?

Most people with angina experience it as a severe, crushing or constricting pain across the front of the chest. It may be described as 'like a band' or 'a heavy weight'. It may radiate through to the back or up into the neck. It is often frightening. It lasts a few minutes and is relieved by rest or nitrates.

A large minority describe it differently: 'not a pain; more a sort of tightness; an uncomfortable feeling'. For many, it is not in the chest at all but in the arms (one or both), fingers, neck, jaw or shoulders. Some describe it as a tingling feeling in the hands or fingers. If it comes on during exercise, it usually forces the person to stop, although some people can 'walk through it'.

When does it happen?

Typically, angina occurs during exercise, eating or emotional stress. It may, however, seem inconsistent, so that the patient can at one time undertake easily an activity which, on another occasion, brings on severe symptoms. There is often another factor, such as fatigue, cold weather or recent food intake to explain the difference. Sometimes precipitating causes overlap: getting angry during a meal, exercise after eating.

Atypical angina, sometimes known as vasospastic angina, occurs at night or at rest. It is more common in women.

Is it angina?

The diagnosis is usually made on the history and in a typical case (see Table 4.2D) is immediately beyond doubt. However, it is not at all unusual for there to be considerable difficulty in coming to a conclusion. The following factors add weight to the diagnosis:

complaint of associated rapid palpitations;
strong family history of ischaemic heart disease under 60;
previous history of myocardial infarction;
known hypertension;
smoking;
general fatigue or recent loss of drive.

What else could it be?

The differential diagnosis is often difficult. It is impossible to prove that anyone does not have angina, even using the most sophisticated diagnostic techniques. However, it is important to try to be as certain as possible. Whilst recognising the importance of not missing the diagnosis, it must be remembered that both the diagnosis and its treatment have devastating and life-long implications and must not be made lightly.

Conditions which may cause confusion:

oesophagitis	pericarditis
gastritis	prodromal herpes zoster
biliary disease	cardiac neurosis
costochondral pain	spinal derangement: neck; upper dorsal spine
anxiety.	

The most useful clues can be obtained by taking a careful history. Most of these conditions do not cause the usually clearly defined pain of angina, closely linked to exertion. They are more likely to grumble on, causing niggling, irritating pain, rather than anything sudden, severe or frightening. Table 4.2D shows the characteristics of chest pain from different causes.

The following symptoms are *unlikely* to be associated with angina:
nausea
dysphagia (especially with hot liquids)
cough
pain relieved by antacids
pain related to breathing
pain related to movement.

Diagnostic pitfalls

Dyspepsia is often relieved by nitrates. Oesophageal spasm is improved by nifedipine as well as by nitrates. Nervous or neurotic individuals are as likely as anyone else to develop ischaemic heart disease. Patients with rapidly increasing symptoms may be about to infarct: unstable or crescendo angina or pre-infarction syndrome.

Table 4.2D Characteristics of chest pain

Chest pain	Angina	Oesophagitis	Musculoskeletal
Where is it?	Retrosternal	Epigastric and retrosternal	Side of chest
Where does it go?	Throat, jaw, ears, arms and hands	Throat, back	Round to front and back
What is it like?	Tight band across chest Heavy, crushing Lasts 5 – 10 minutes	Burning Often prolonged	Sharp, spasms or constant ache
What brings it on?	Exertion Heavy meal	Swallowing, especially hot fluids Bending down	Movement of chest shoulders or neck
What makes it better?	Rest GTN	Antacids GTN	Change in position Rest Analgesics
Previous history?	Ischaemic heart disease Myocardial infarction Hypertension	Dyspepsia	Backache Stiff neck

Hyperventilation is a sign of anxiety and tension but itself may precipitate or exacerbate angina in a susceptible individual. It may also cause non-cardiac chest pain which may be difficult to interpret.

What do you find?

Coronary atheroma, on its own, produces no physical signs and so examination of patients with angina often reveals nothing. However, sometimes an important, remediable, precipitating condition is found. Therefore, it is of the utmost importance that these patients should be examined carefully and thoroughly.

Look for evidence:

(1)   which tends to confirm the diagnosis, or point to other conditions which might have precipitated the angina or be contributing to it, e.g:

arcus senilis	aortic stenosis
xantholasma	diabetes
tendon xanthomata	hypertension
cardiac arrhythmia	hyperthyroidism
heart failure	anaemia.

(2)   which tends to support an alternative diagnosis, such as:
           pain on movement of spine (especially the neck)
           costochondral tenderness
           epigastric tenderness
           jaundice
           hyperaesthesia (or rash) of herpes zoster.

What investigations?

Every patient, in whom angina is suspected, should have the following investigations:
    ECG
    chest X-ray
    full blood count
    blood sugar
    urine test for glucose, albumen and cells.
If there is the slightest suspicion of hyperthyroidism then thyroid function tests should be done. It is easy to miss this in the elderly, in whom the classical symptoms and signs are often absent (forme fruste).
    A lipoprotein profile should be done in the young and may be useful even in the elderly if there is a younger generation who may be at risk.

What might these investigations show?

They may all be normal. This would in no way exclude the diagnosis.

(1)   *The ECG* may be normal or it may show evidence of diffuse ischaemia with (see Figures 4.2F, 4.2G) flattened S – T segments or misshapen or inverted T waves in some leads; of previous myocardial infarction; of LVH suggestive of other disease (e.g. hypertension, aortic stenosis) or of arrhythmia.

(2)   *Chest X-ray* is likely to be normal but it may show evidence of cardiac abnormality (hypertrophy, ventricular aneurysm), of heart failure, pericardial effusion or coarctation of the aorta.

(3)   *Full blood count* may show evidence of anaemia.

(4)   *Blood sugar* may suggest, or confirm, diabetes.

(5)   *Lipoprotein profile* may reveal hyperlipidaemia.

(6)   *Urine test* may show evidence of renal disease.

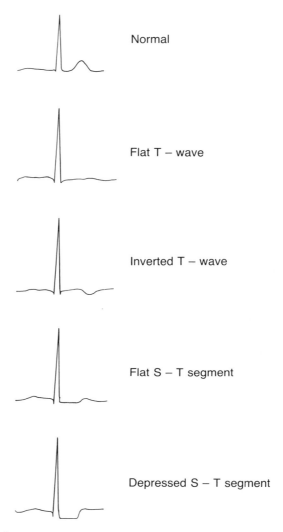

Figure 4.2F ECG changes

What does the diagnosis of angina mean?

In the majority of people with angina, it can be taken as evidence of coronary atheroma. (There may be some, with vasospastic angina, in whom the coronary arteries are normal.) 14% become symptom free and live for many years. 20% will be dead within 5 years (4% per annum).

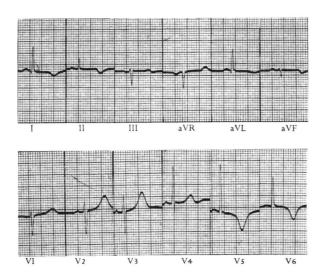

I II III aVR aVL aVF

VI V2 V3 V4 V5 V6

Figure 4.2G Ischaemic ECG (see also Figure 3.5K, p.127)

It is impossible to give an accurate prognosis in any particular individual: short-term, intermediate or long-term. Patients with angina, like those without, may have a fatal myocardial infarct or arrhythmia at any time. Alternatively, they may live for many years with varying degrees of disability. Most can expect reasonable control of their symptoms for a considerable period without intolerable side-effects from the drugs. They should be encouraged to lead normal lives. It is therefore possible to be both honest and encouraging to the individual.

Management

> Crescendo angina, when symptoms are increasing
> in frequency or severity, may presage an
> imminent infarct and should be treated urgently,
> preferably by admission to hospital.

In the non-urgent situation, management must first be directed towards treating any remediable contributory condition, such as hypertension (see above).

For the angina itself, the management can be divided into General (non-drug) measures; Drug treatment; Surgery and Follow-up.

General measures

If the onset of symptoms is recent, the patient should have an initial period of rest at home, while the situation is being assessed and the drug regime established.

Look at the overall situation. If the patient lives with another adult, it is helpful to see both together so that a realistic strategy can be planned which has a good chance of being implemented.

Discuss the condition: what it is, what it means, what it does not mean. Has he or she any particular fears? His father or a brother may have dropped dead at his age or a friend may recently have had a heart attack. He maybe anxious about his own future, about his family, his job, about money. Anxiety is likely to aggravate the symptoms and make them more difficult to treat. It is, therefore, well worth while devoting some time to discussion and explanation. Most people with angina are well and active for many years after the diagnosis. It does not mean that he is about to have a heart attack. His symptoms can be successfully treated.

Discuss details of the symptom: its pattern in relation to daily life, things which bring it on, how it can be avoided.

Discuss life-style: smoking must stop – at once/no argument although help and support need not be denied. The partner should be asked to give up too. Relationships may need to be examined: it may be possible to lessen friction and ease tension. Is it possible for this person to become more relaxed?

Exercise is important as it encourages the development of collaterals as well as improving fitness, lessening the work the heart has to do and being good for morale.

It should be taken sensibly, within the limitations of the symptom and increased gradually over an extended period as fitness develops. Intense exertion, like squash, should be avoided as it is associated with an increased incidence of sudden death. It is important for the patient to work out for himself what he can do and not to depend on the doctor to give instructions. One of the most devastating aspects of being faced with the diagnosis of angina is the feeling of helplessness and dependency that is often engendered. The quality of life can be greatly improved if the patient is able to realise that he is still in charge of his own actions.

Sexual activity is usually unaffected but some people may be afraid to try. It has been reported that extramarital sex is more likely to be associated with sudden death. Some anti-anginal drugs, especially beta-blockers, cause impotence. Everyone should be encouraged to continue normally.

Diet may have to change. It is important for anyone with angina to be slim for the obvious reason that the heart has less work to do than in someone who is obese. It is also usual to advise a diet low in saturated fats (see p.327), although it is not established that the atheromatous process can be reversed at this stage.

Discuss work: most people can continue with the same work but people with any evidence of ischaemic heart disease are excluded from some jobs. These include pilots and those needing an HGV licence. If the work is physically very strenuous, then it may be necessary to seek a change to a lighter job. Excessively long hours are best avoided and so is a great deal of travelling. Some companies are very helpful in meeting the person's needs, others, less so. Sometimes, a letter or telephone call from the doctor helps (with the patient's permission).

Discuss when to seek medical advice: IMMEDIATELY if an acute attack is not relieved by rest and medication within an hour; SOON if the attacks are not well controlled or are increasing in frequency or severity.

Provide written information to confirm, amplify and reiterate the advice.

Drug treatment

Medication in angina is used for the relief of symptoms. It does not appear to influence the prognosis. The aim is to increase coronary perfusion or to reduce myocardial oxygen requirements or both.

Coronary perfusion can be increased by dilating the coronary arteries (e.g. with nitrates or calcium antagonists), and by allowing more time for coronary blood flow. This means slowing the heart to extend diastole, which is when the coronary flow takes place, e.g. with beta-blockers.

Myocardial oxygen requirements can be reduced by reducing the work load of the heart. This can be achieved by rest; by reducing venous return to the heart (e.g. with nitrates, which cause dilatation of peripheral veins); by reducing the peripheral resistance by using drugs which dilate systemic arteries (e.g. nifedipine); by reducing heart rate (e.g. with beta-blockers); and by reducing contractility (e.g. with beta-blockers or calcium-channel blockers).

Often, the best effects are obtained by using combinations of drugs.

Figures 4.2H and 4.2I present a physiological model showing where drugs act.

Drugs may not be needed if the general measures, outlined above, are effective. However, it is a good policy to advise all patients to take aspirin 75 mg daily (to reduce platelet stickiness and the risk of infarction) and to carry a short-acting nitrate (to increase confidence, at least to start with, until he has learnt how his angina is going to behave).

Anti-anginal drugs can be considered under the following headings.

(1)	Nitrates: short-acting long-acting	(3)	Calcium-channel blockers
(2)	Beta-blocker	(4)	Combined treatment

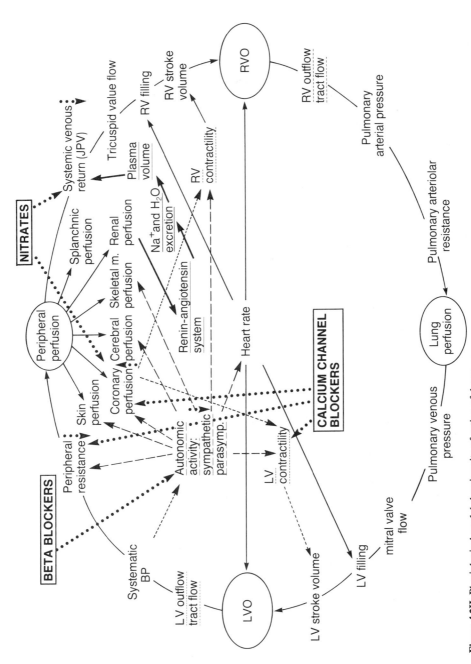

Figure 4.2H Physiological model showing site of action of drugs

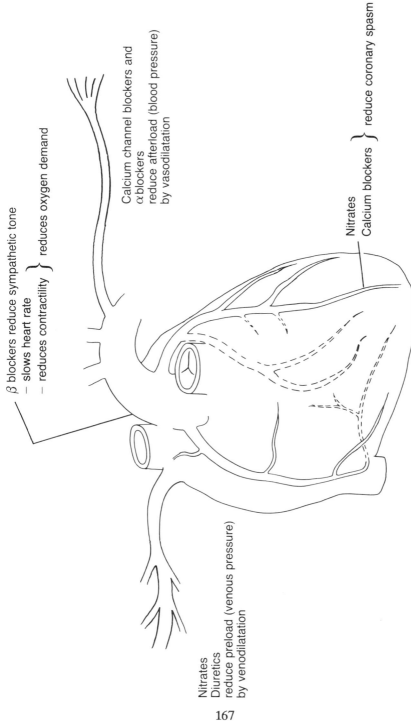

β blockers reduce sympathetic tone
− slows heart rate
− reduces contractility } reduces oxygen demand

Calcium channel blockers and
α blockers
reduce afterload (blood pressure)
by vasodilatation

Nitrates
Calcium blockers } reduce coronary spasm

Nitrates
Diuretics
reduce preload (venous pressure)
by venodilatation

Figure 4.2I Drawing of heart showing site of action of drugs

(1)   **Nitrates** dilate the coronary arteries and systemic veins, improving coronary blood flow, reducing the workload of the heart and increasing exercise tolerance.

Short-acting nitrates for use when angina occurs or for short-term prevention.

(i) glyceryl trinitrate (GTN):
  − tablets: 500 mcg sublingually (300 mcg tablets are available for anyone who is intolerant of the larger dose);
  − spray: 400 mcg per metered dose sublingually. (The dose can be repeated every 3 min until the pain goes, up to a maximum of four tablets or doses of spray);
  − slow-release tablets (Suscard): 1−2 mg. These are placed between upper lip and gum and left to dissolve.

(ii)   isosorbide dinitrate tablets:
  − 5−10 mg sublingually.

GTN tablets and spray begin to work within 1 to 2 min and last from 30 min to 1 h. The other preparations act within 5 min and continue for about 8 h.

All these drugs are most effective when used immediately before the onset of the pain. Many patients become adept at this, finding the angina quite predictable. For others, it is more difficult.

If used to treat an attack, the patient should stop and sit down to take the drug. If he lies down, the venous return to the heart is increased. This increases the workload and so makes the angina worse. If he remains standing he may faint as a result of the reduced cardiac output caused by the (intended) reduction in venous return to the heart resulting from veno-dilatation.

Short-acting nitrates are especially liable to cause headache, flushing and faintness from postural hypotension. These problems may by avoided by starting with a small dose and gradually increasing it as tolerance to the side-effects develops.Some people are never able to tolerate them. Of these, some can take long-acting nitrates and others have to be treated with a different group of drugs altogether.

Long-acting nitrates used for preventing angina:

(i)   isosorbide mononitrate: 5−40 mg, twice or three times a day;

(ii)   isosorbide dinitrate: 5−40 mg, twice or three times a day;

(iii)   slow-release glyceryl trinitrate: 1–10 mg, depending on the preparation used, twice or three times a day;

(iv)   self-adhesive skin patches: one every 24 h.

Long-acting nitrates appear to offer a tremendous advantage over other forms of medication in people who can tolerate them.

The main doubt about their use centres on the question of whether their effect is sustained during prolonged treatment or whether tolerance develops. It seems likely that some degree of tolerance does develop and that this may seriously reduce the effectiveness of the drug in some people. High doses and continuous treatment appear to make this problem worse and so it is worth trying to find the lowest dose which is effective and to build a nitrate-free period into the regimen, for instance by giving the last dose in the early evening.

Isosorbide mononitrate gives more consistent results than the dinitrate because it is itself the active drug. The dinitrate is converted to mononitrate by the liver before it is effective and therefore depends on liver function.

Skin patches have not been proved to have a reliably sustained effect.

All nitrates should be stored, as far as possible, according to the manufacturers instructions. This is a problem for many people: the greatest need for short-acting nitrates is when out and about and men usually carry them in a trouser pocket. Here, they are warm and GTN tablets deteriorate rapidly.

(For more details, see Chapter 2.3 p.67).

(2)   **Beta-blockers** are the mainstay of treatment of angina in patients who can tolerate them and in whom they are no contra-indications (see p.59). They reduce oxygen requirements by slowing the heart and reducing contractility (negative inotropic effect).

All beta-blockers are equally effective in preventing angina. They do so in about 80% of patients. They are not effective in atypical (Prinzmetal's) angina.

The choice depends on which drug the doctor is used to prescribing; the incidence of side-effects; the length of action; the presence of a complicating condition, such as hypertension or arrhythmia, and on the need for a cardioselective drug.

It may be advisable to avoid those with partial agonist activity as they do not reduce the heart rate so effectively, especially during exercise.

Propranolol has been widely used in the past and there is no reason to stop anyone taking it, if it suits them. However, it has numerous disadvantages: it is not cardioselective and is more likely to cause bronchospasm and problems with the peripheral circulation; it is lipid soluble and passes the blood–brain barrier freely, producing central side-effects; it has a high first pass metabolism and therefore an unpredictable effect for a given dose and it is short-acting and needs to be taken three to four times a day unless a long-acting preparation is used.

(3)   **Calcium-channel blockers** are useful in patients who cannot take beta-blockers and in those who need maximal (triple) therapy – see below. They relieve angina by dilating the coronary arteries, reducing peripheral resistance (afterload) and therefore cardiac work and by reducing contractility (negative inotropic effect) which reduces oxygen requirements. They must not be given to patients with significant aortic stenosis.

(4)   *Combined treatment* – a combination of two, or even three, types of drugs is often effective when one alone fails to control symptoms.

(i)   Nitrates and beta-blockers: both these groups of drugs decrease the workload, and, therefore, the oxygen requirements, of the heart. Nitrates also increase coronary blood flow. They are complementary, each tending to cancel out some of the undesirable effects of the other:
- nitrates cause tachycardia, beta-blockers, bradycardia;
- beta-blockers increase heart size, nitrates reduce it;
- beta-blockers reduce peripheral perfusion, nitrates increase it. They therefore make a useful combination for many people. They should be used with care in heart failure (see p.59).

(ii)   Nitrates and calcium antagonists: this combination is especially likely to be effective in vasospastic and atypical angina and, therefore, in women. Nifedipine is the calcium antagonist most usually prescribed but verapamil and diltiazem are equally effective.

(iii)   Nitrates, beta-blockers and calcium antagonists: triple therapy. Increasing the number of drugs to three, does not necessarily mean a more powerful effect and there is a possibility of inducing hypotension. However, they may be helpful when maximal therapy is needed. Care is needed if there is a risk of heart failure. Verapamil should not be given with a beta-blocker.

Typical regime for maximal triple therapy of angina

Isosorbide mononitrate: 20 mg three times daily
Atenolol: 100 mg once daily
Nifedipine S.R: 20 mg twice daily
GTN spray prn

Care should be taken to avoid prescribing more than one drug from the same group. If a beta-blocker is not having the desired effect, then the dose may be increased or the drug changed. There is no point in adding another beta-blocker and it might cause serious problems. The same applies to the other groups of drugs.

If a new drug is prescribed, the patient must understand whether it is to be taken instead of, or as well as, those he is currently taking.

Why does angina sometimes get worse again despite medication?

(1)   The disease process may have extended:
       – a reappraisal of the whole situation is called for.

(2)   Nitrate tolerance may have developed:
       – an increase in dose or different combination may help.
       – a nitrate-free period of 8 hours or more increases efficacy.

(3)   The drugs may not be used as advised:
       – out of date:
           – the patient may not realise that nitrates deteriorate;
           – may feel they should not be 'wasted' (i.e. replaced when few have been used);
       – erratic dosage:
           – 'trying to manage without';
           – 'I don't want to get used to them'.

(4)   Heart failure may have developed:
       – this makes angina more resistant to conventional treatment. If it is recognised and treated, the angina becomes easier to control.

(5)   There may be an arrhythmia:
       – an ECG or 24-hour tape may be needed.

Surgery

Surgery is most suitable for patients with localised stenoses of the main coronary arteries (see Figure 1.2E in Chapter 1.2). It cannot benefit those in whom the narrowing is peripheral. This is more likely to be the case in women and in diabetics.

In coronary artery bypass grafting (see Figure 4.2J), a length of the patients own long saphenous vein or internal mammary artery is used. Coronary artery bypass grafting improves the prognosis for the following

171

groups of patients:
- those with localised stenosis of the left main stem coronary artery;
- those with proximal three-vessel disease: circumflex, left anterior descending (LAD) and right coronary arteries;
- those with poor left ventricular function.

In coronary angioplasty (Figure 4.2K), a balloon catheter is passed via the femoral artery into the affected coronary artery to the point of maximum constriction and inflated. This crushes the plaque and opens up the lumen of the artery.

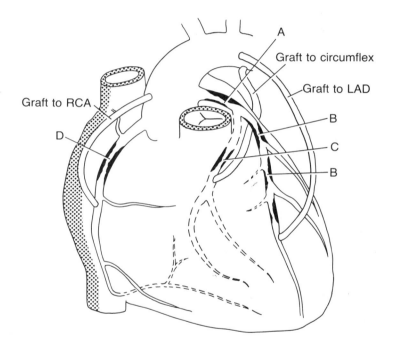

Figure 4.2J Common sites of stenosis due to coronary atheroma and positions of bypass grafts
A = Main stem of left coronary artery
B = Left anterior descending (LAD)
C = Circumflex
D = Right coronary artery (RCA)

In terms of relief of symptoms, the results of these procedures, in suitable patients, are good. The procedures offer less prospect of success in women.

In an ideal situation, anyone with angina should be offered referral for assessment of the possible benefits of surgery, unless they are obviously unsuitable because of advanced age or intercurrent disease.

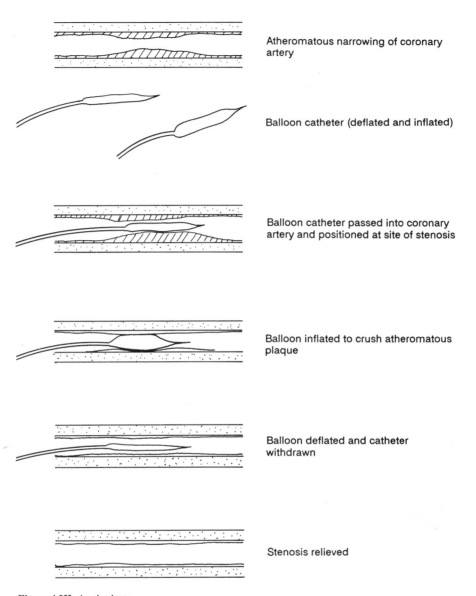

Atheromatous narrowing of coronary artery

Balloon catheter (deflated and inflated)

Balloon catheter passed into coronary artery and positioned at site of stenosis

Balloon inflated to crush atheromatous plaque

Balloon deflated and catheter withdrawn

Stenosis relieved

Figure 4.2K Angioplasty

In practice, in the UK, surgical intervention is, at present, offered only to people with severe symptoms which do not respond to medical treatment or who are under 50 and have severe anatomical disease irrespective of symptoms.

173

Follow-up

The drugs used in the treatment of angina are powerful, variable in effect, capable of causing unpleasant side-effects or of losing altogether the beneficial effect they had to start with.

In addition, the underlying process of coronary atheroma may progress to cause more severe angina, myocardial infarction or heart failure or all of these.

Not all of these problems will be obvious to the patient, who may well have only a sketchy idea of the nature of his disease and its treatment. He or she is certainly unlikely to understand the actions and interactions of the various drugs he is taking.

It is, therefore, of the utmost importance for follow-up to be meticulous, regular and life-long. (For suggestions as to how this may be organised, see Chapter 5.3 p.324.)

How often the patient is seen will depend on a number of factors: the severity of the symptoms, the stability of the disease, the success of the treatment, the level of understanding of the patient and the complexity of the drug regime.

Follow-up will need to be at frequent intervals, at first; less often later, if the condition is stable. Its purpose is to monitor the control of symptoms; the appearance of new symptoms; adherence to advice: smoking, diet, weight reduction; self-confidence and adjustment; ability to cope with work; weight; blood pressure and pulse; use of drugs and social adjustment.

These visits provide an opportunity to watch for the development of crescendo angina: increasing frequency, severity or length of attacks, which may warn of impending infarction; early symptoms of heart failure: breathlessness on exertion, orthopnoea, nocturnal cough, paroxysmal nocturnal dyspnoea, oedema and for symptoms or signs of arrhythmia: palpitations, fits, faints, falls or dizzy turns.

Who to refer?

The reasons for making a referral to a cardiologist are in the hope that he or she will be able to confirm or refute the diagnosis where it is in doubt; confirm or exclude complicating conditions; identify patients in whom surgery may be helpful (coronary artery bypass graft or angioplasty) and advise on treatment, if necessary.

It is therefore useful to refer the following patients:

(1)   Those in whom it is difficult to make a definite diagnosis or in whom there are puzzling or inconsistent findings suggestive of an uncommon condition, such as a cardiomyopathy.

(2)   Those in whom valvular disease is suspected, especially aortic stenosis.

(3)   Those with complex arrhythmias or in whom arrhythmias are suspected on the history, even if not confirmed on ECG.

(4)   Anyone under 60.

(5)   Those who fail to respond to treatment.

What will the cardiologist do?

He or she will confirm the diagnosis, if necessary carrying out further tests, such as an exercise test; identify any complicating factors; recommend changes in medical treatment; and identify and investigate anyone likely to benefit from surgery. This will usually include exercise testing and angiography. (Remember that even a cardiologist, with all the most sophisticated equipment, cannot prove that a patient does *not* have angina.)

175

4.2.5   MYOCARDIAL INFARCTION

What is it?

It is the death of heart muscle due to obstruction of a coronary artery.

Whom does it affect?

In a practice population of 2,000, six patients will suffer myocardial infarction (MI) every year. Of these, three will die suddenly, three will be under 65 years and two will never reach retirement age.

What causes it?

Ischaemic heart disease: a coronary artery, narrowed by atheroma, becomes totally blocked by the formation of a thrombus.

Spasm of a partially occluded artery may be an important additional precipitating factor, especially during intense exercise, like playing squash.

What happens?

There is a sudden reduction of coronary perfusion, with complete block of flow to a part of the myocardium. This has an effect on the whole myocardium and not only on the part which has had its blood supply cut off.

There is an immediate reduction in contractility. The results of this are more devastating than happens when the ischaemic process develops gradually over an extended period, allowing compensatory mechanisms time to come into play.

Stroke volume, especially that of the left ventricle, falls, immediately reducing cardiac output. This leads to a fall in blood pressure and very rapid increase in sympathetic tone. This, in turn, causes an increase in heart rate and in contractility of any myocardium capable of responding. This increases the oxygen requirements of the heart – which can only be supplied by the increase in coronary perfusion that is not available. The increased sympathetic tone has an adverse effect on the heart, which is already struggling to maintain an adequate output with decreased perfusion.

Arrhythmias are common. A tachyarrhythmia embarrasses the heart by reducing time for coronary perfusion at the same time as causing an increased need for oxygen. It also reduces stroke volume (and therefore cardiac output) by reducing filling time. Bradyarrhythmias reduce cardiac output by slowing the heart.

Within a short time, the reduction in cardiac output and of peripheral perfusion, including renal perfusion, stimulates the renin–angiotensin system. This causes both increases in peripheral arteriolar tone, and therefore of peripheral resistance (afterload), and also of sodium and water retention and plasma volume. Both these effects increase the work load of the heart and are unhelpful.

The physiological model is perturbed as shown in Figure 4.2L.

Half of all deaths occur immediately but when someone dies suddenly it is often impossible to determine an exact cause of death, even with a post mortem examination. If there is no clear cause, a label of sudden cardiac death (SCD) is usually applied. This usually means cardiac arrest due to ventricular fibrillation or, less commonly, asystole. Acute coronary occlusion is often the precipitating factor. The risk of death is not necessarily related to the degree of coronary artery disease nor to the size of the infarct. Muscle death does not occur for an hour or more after the blood supply is cut off but acutely ischaemic myocardium is irritable and arrhythmias are common immediately after a coronary artery is obstructed.

Myocardial infarction may present as sudden death with little or no warning; as severe, continuous, crushing, retrosternal pain, possibly radiating into the neck, jaw, arms, back or as the rapid or gradual onset of symptoms and signs of heart failure without significant chest pain: the 'silent infarct'. This is especially common in the elderly.

In any of these situations, the patient may have had a period of angina, either for the first time or increasing in frequency or severity (crescendo angina) during the previous days or weeks.

It is also common for an acute infarct to be preceded by a feeling of weariness and general malaise (the pre-infarction syndrome).

What do you find?

> Obvious severe pain
> Fear
> Pallor
> Shock: skin cold, sweating
> Tachycardia (sometimes, bradycardia: see below).

The blood pressure may be:

(1)   low because cardiac output is reduced;

(2)   normal because heart is coping well or because the patient was previously hypertensive but now has a reduced cardiac output (decapitated hypertension);

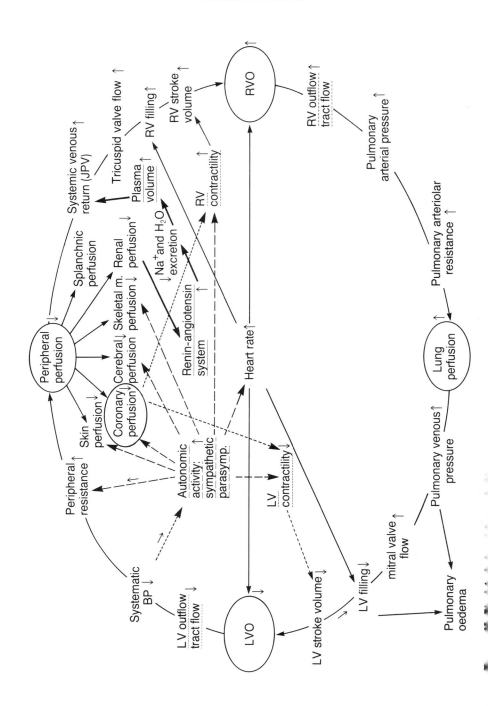

(3)   high because of pre-existing hypertension or because increased
       sympathetic activity resulting from pain, fear or homeostatic
       mechanism (see Figure 1.3J) is overwhelming the tendency for the
       cardiac output to fall.

Is it myocardial infarction?

If classical symptoms and signs are present, then treatment should begin at
once, before a definitive diagnosis is attempted.

The ECG

In the acute phase, a normal ECG does not exclude a diagnosis of myocardial
infarction. There may be non-specific S–T segment and T wave changes
suggesting ischaemia but classical signs of infarction may not appear for up to
3 days.

   If there are no diagnostic ECG changes (see below), repeat the ECG
later and rely on the cardiac enzymes meanwhile.

   Over the affected area of myocardium, the ECG tracing will change as
shown in Figure 4.2M.

First few hours: normal [± old changes]
                  OR
                  S–T segments elevated and peaked T waves.

12–24 hours: S–T segments elevated
                  pathological q waves
                  T waves becoming inverted.

Next few days: S–T segments return to base line
                  q waves persist.

Later: T waves more noticeably inverted
                  T wave inversion may persist OR become upright
                  Q waves usually persist.

S–T segments and T waves usually remain permanently distorted to some
extent.

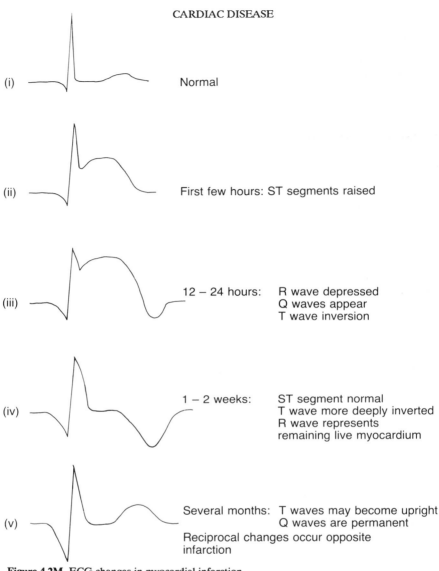

(i) Normal

(ii) First few hours: ST segments raised

(iii) 12 – 24 hours: R wave depressed
Q waves appear
T wave inversion

(iv) 1 – 2 weeks: ST segment normal
T wave more deeply inverted
R wave represents
remaining live myocardium

(v) Several months: T waves may become upright
Q waves are permanent
Reciprocal changes occur opposite
infarction

Figure 4.2M ECG changes in myocardial infarction

Site of the infarct

(1) Anterior (left coronary artery):
  – changes in leads V1–6 i.e. those which reflect electrical activity in the anterior part of the heart (left ventricle);
  – this is more likely to lead to LVF or left ventricular aneurysm.

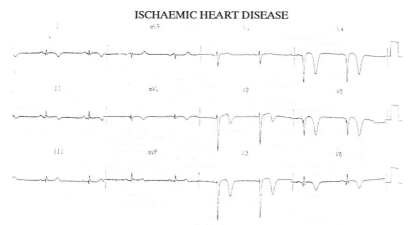

Figure 4.2N ECG in acute antero-septal myocardial infarction

(2)   Posterior or inferior (right coronary artery):
   –   changes in leads II, III and aVf;
   –   more likely to cause arrhythmias because conducting tissue is damaged.

ECG changes are shown in Figures 4.2N and 4.2O.

Cardiac enzymes

These are released from damaged myocardial cells.
   Increased serum levels are seen (Figure 4.2P) for:
   –   creatinine phosphokinase (CPK) – max. at 16 h;
   –   alanine serum transaminase (AST or SGOT) – max. at 24 h;
   –   lactic dehydrogenase (LDH) – max. at 72 h.

The serum levels of these enzymes may also be raised in other circumstances:

(1)   LDH in the presence of skeletal muscle damage and pulmonary embolism;
(2)   AST (SGOT) if there is hepatocellular damage;
(3)   Both in severe pulmonary oedema.

181

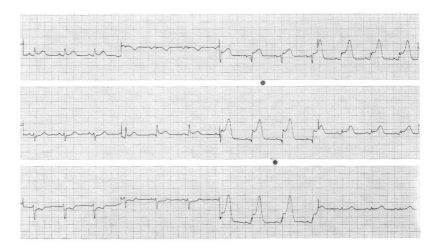

Figure 4.2O ECG in acute anterior myocardial infarction (early)

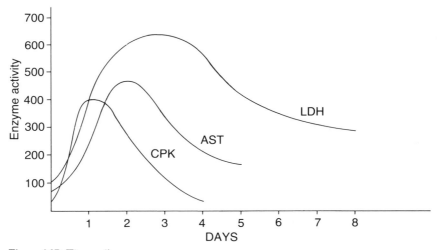

Figure 4.2P The cardiac enzymes

What else might it be?

Pulmonary embolism

- This may be impossible to distinguish from myocardial infarction.
- Small emboli cause pleuritic pain, disproportionate breathlessness and occasionally, haemoptysis.

182

- An apparent source may suggest the diagnosis:
  - tender calf
  - recent pelvic or leg operation or fracture.

Spontaneous pneumothorax

- Affects younger age group
- There is pain to one side: lacks the severe, crushing, frightening quality of the classical myocardial infarction (MI) although this may be absent even in the presence of infarction (see above).
- There is marked breathlessness.
- Air entry is reduced over the upper lobe on the side affected.

Dissecting aneurysm

- This causes pain similar to acute MI but starts suddenly.
- Pain often radiates to back; may have a 'tearing' quality.
- Peripheral pulses may be absent or unequal.
- Aortic systolic murmur may appear.

Hysteria and cardiac neurosis

- Symptoms settle after a few minutes quiet conversation.
- The patient is easily distracted and able to talk fluently, using long sentences: good breath control in marked contrast to the distressed patient with acute MI.
- May be superimposed on another non-cardiac condition, such as costochondritis.

Oesophagitis

- Previous history is an indicator.
- Worse after food (especially hot fluids).
- Relieved by antacids
- Nitrates may give relief.

Cholecystitis

- Previous history is an indicator.

– Fat intolerance, nausea, vomiting occur.
– Murphy's sign is positive.

Herpes zoster

– Pain may precede the rash by several days.
– Hyperaesthesia may be marked.

Pericarditis

– Pain varies with position and with respiration.
– Rub best heard with patient leaning forward and exhaling.

Thoracic root pain

– Is worse with movement.
– Is relieved by lying flat.

What should you do?

Give immediately:
(1) Sublingual GTN (spray should be carried in the doctor's bag).
(2) Pain relief – is urgent and has a clear influence on the outcome.

PAIN RELIEF

Diamorphine 5 mg

WITH   STAT; i.v.; SLOWLY (over 3 min)

Cyclizine 25 mg

1. These can be conveniently administered by dissolving 10 mg diamorphine in a 1 ml ampoule of cyclizine (50 mg) and giving half of the resulting solution.
2. If this does not control the pain, half of what is left can be given and the rest 10 min later, if the pain is still persisting.
3. Aged, frail or lightweight patients should be given half of this dosage.

Note that:

− Respiratory depression is a serious risk and larger doses should be avoided, unless the pain persists for a reasonable interval after the injection is completed.

− Administration by the i.m. or s.c. routes should be avoided: the peripheral circulation may be reduced; uptake delayed; the expected immediate effect needed not achieved; the dose is repeated and respiratory depression later is a real risk. Patients often reach hospital in a state of respiratory depression, following this sequence of events.

− Naloxone: 200−400 mcg should be available for i.v. use in case of respiratory depression.

(3)   Antithrombotic agents: aspirin, half a tablet (150 mg). Thrombolytic agents may soon be in general use.

Complications

(1)   Bradycardia: 50/ min or less affects about 20% of patients:

− Give atropine: 300−600 mcg; i.v., SLOWLY;
  − repeat every 10 min until pulse rate rises (60−80);
  − maximum 1800 mcg (three ampoules of 600 mcg each);
  − beware of giving too much.

(2)   Tachycardia: it is usual for anyone who has just had an acute MI to have an increased pulse rate, as a result of pain and fear, even if there is no heart failure or arrhythmia.
       If the heart rate is persistently over 140/min and it is not possible to obtain an ECG immediately, then it must be assumed that this is ventricular tachycardia and should be treated with lignocaine:

− Give lignocaine: 100 mg; i.v., SLOWLY. Pause after 50 mg in elderly.

(3)   Breathlessness: may indicate acute LVF and, in an emergency, has to be treated as such:

− Give frusemide: 20 mg; i.v., SLOWLY.

(4)   Collapse: no radial or carotid pulse.

- Assume that this is due to cardiac arrest due to ventricular fibrillation or asystole.
- Resuscitation is worth attempting (see Table 4.2C, p.153) if you arrive within 10 min of the collapse, as it is impossible to say when the circulation actually stopped.
  - strike a blow on the lower sternum if you witness the collapse;
  - give external cardiac massage;
  - clear airway and start mouth-to-mouth or mouth-to-nose respiration;
  - send for coronary ambulance.

What happens next?

Consider hospital or home care.

Hospital admission

(1)   Advantages:
        Coronary care facilities – monitoring, resuscitation team in case of cardiac arrest or serious arrhythmia, thrombolysis;
        Nursing care continuously available;
        Possible reduction of anxiety in patient and relatives.

(2)   Disadvantages:
        Journey may precipitate disastrous arrhythmia;
        Coronary care facilities may be unavailable;
        Staff are unfamiliar;
        Hospital may be understaffed, nurses scarce and overall care inadequate;
        Ward may be crowded, noisy, frightening and depressing.

Home care

(1)   Advantages:
        Quiet, restful, familiar surroundings;
        Avoids journey;
        Familiar carers – family, doctor, district nurse.

(2)   Disadvantages:
        No resuscitation facilities;
        Possibly less medical expertise.

Factors to consider

There is no clear guidance from statistical studies: the evidence is conflicting. Doctors have to advise the patient on an individual basis, taking into account both the overall local provision in terms of hospital and community services and their own level of expertise as well as the circumstances of the particular patient.

If there is a policy worked out with the local physicians, then this is of considerable importance.

The risk of serious arrhythmia is highest during the first few hours. After that, it reduces rapidly.

Questions to ask

(1)   Is the journey likely to be delayed, long or especially disturbing?

(2)   Is the patient at high risk of arrhythmia, bradycardia, tachycardia (on initial examination), irregular pulse or multiple ventricular ectopics on ECG, previous history of arrhythmia?

(3)   What are the home circumstances?
           Does he live alone or with a frail relative?
           Is there a telephone in the house?
           Is a district nurse available?
           Can the doctor attend easily and at short notice?
           What are the arrangements for medical cover out of hours?
           Where is the patient? . . . if downstairs, can he be nursed there; is
           there a downstairs WC or commode available and acceptable?
           What does the patient want to do? It is ultimately his decision,
           whatever the doctor thinks and he is likely to make better progress,
           if his wishes are respected.
           What do the relatives want?

(4)   Is the local hospital reasonably near and well staffed and equipped with full coronary care facilities available to patients in this age group? (In some hospitals, full care is not available to those over 65 years.)

The choices to be considered are set out in Table 4.2E.

Table 4.2E Myocardial infarction: home or hospital?

Home	Hospital
Low risk	*High risk*
Pain more than 6 hours ago	Pain less than 4 hours ago
No pain now	Pain continuing
Not breathless	Breathless
Pulse regular and normal rate	Arrhythmia
BP satisfactory	BP low: shocked
Long journey to hospital	
Other factors	
Age of patient	Telephone
Patient choice	Hospital facilities
Family choice/attitudes	Help available: spouse, family,
House accessible	community nurse

Admission to hospital

Having considered all the factors, most patients under 70 will be admitted to hospital, unless they are first seen more than 6 hours after the pain has stopped and are stable.

(1)   Ask for a 'coronary' ambulance for the journey, if one is available.

(2)   Make sure pain relief is as effective as possible.

(3)   Give emergency treatment for arrhythmia or heart failure, if necessary.

(4)   Provide as much information as possible in the accompanying letter. The house physician is unlikely to remember what he or she is told on the telephone and if the admission is arranged through a bed service, little useful information will arrive at the hospital with the patient.

The following are important:
– immediate history;
– details of drugs given;
– details of observations, such as pulse rate and BP;
– previous history of heart disease, ECG findings (including whether a recent ECG has been normal);
– details of recent drugs and especially of sensitivities;
– details of any relevant previous admissions to hospital.

Home care

(1)   Examination:
  - General condition including:
      pain
      breathlessness
      orthopnoea
      colour
      anxiety level.
  - Radial pulse: rate, rhythm, equal at both wrists?
  - Femoral pulse: if delayed or difficult to find – dissecting aneurysm?
  - Blood pressure: compare with previous readings, if known.
  - Lungs: are there rales and rhonchi, which might confirm left heart failure? Do not attach too much importance to basal creps: they are common and usually insignificant.
  - JVP; liver; sacral or ankle oedema.

(2)   Investigations:
  - ECG:
      - as soon as possible;
      - repeat after 3 days, if inconclusive;
      - repeat at any time, if arrhythmia or extension of infarct suspected;
      - for changes see p.179.
  - Blood for:
      - FBC
      - urea and electrolytes
      - cardiac enzymes
      - thyroid function tests, if appropriate
      - blood sugar.

(3)   The first few days:
  - Pain control continues to be the first consideration.
  - If pain persists, the decision to care for the patient at home should be reconsidered: is the diagnosis correct? is there some unidentified complication such as pericarditis or pulmonary embolism?

(4)   General care:

  - Give reassurance – 'the worst is over'.

- Give an explanation – this should be as full, detailed and oft repeated as the patient needs. This is one of the rare situations in medical practice where it may be advisable to speak to relatives out of the hearing of the patient. It is important that they understand the potential seriousness of the situation and some doctors will wish to place the emphasis of what they say differently when talking to relatives. It may be obvious to the doctor that a sudden, fatal outcome is possible but the family may not appreciate this at all.

- What should the patient do?

  The doctor may think it does not matter very much or that he should do whatever he feels like but patients and relatives usually like to have detailed guidelines and there is no harm in providing them for the first 10 days – after that, see rehabilitation.

  Days 0–3: bed rest: half-sitting, up to commode or WC, in wheel chair. Move feet and legs at frequent intervals.
  Days 4–5: sit out in chair for short periods.
  Days 6–7: walk about room.
  Day 7 and after: use stairs.
  Day 10 and after: short walks outside, weather permitting.

- What can he eat?
  Unrestricted fluids, small quantities of alcohol if liked, light diet if hungry.

(5)   What the doctor should be told about:
      further chest pain of any sort
      breathlessness
      palpitations
      dizzy spells, faints or funny turns
      pain or swelling of legs.

(6)   Watch for symptoms and signs of:

- pericarditis: pleuritic pain with or without fever. Pericardial rub usual but transient.

- heart failure: breathlessness, orthopnoea, paroxysmal nocturnal dyspnoea, raised JVP, enlarged or tender liver, tachycardia, hypotension, 3rd or 4th heart sound.

Tachycardia, without other signs of heart failure, suggests compensated heart failure. This means that the heart can maintain an adequate output only by means of an increased rate. It should be treated because it is a sign that the heart is overloaded and it can quickly develop into fullblown heart failure.

– arrhythmias: palpitations, dizzy spells, faints, angina at rest.

– extension of infarct: recurrent or persistent ischaemic pain.

– DVT.
– emboli: pulmonary or cerebral.

– serious mechanical complications: VSD – pansystolic murmur at LSE with thrill, fall in BP, rise in JVP. Papillary muscle dysfunction – initial regurgitant murmur at apex, no-thrill, increasing SOB, tachycardia.

(7)   Drug treatment:

– for all patients:
    – pain relief as necessary: nitrates or opiates for further ischaemic pain, indomethacin for pericarditis;
    – nitrates (e.g. isosorbide mononitrate 10 mg three times a day);
    – aspirin 75 mg daily.
    – *Note that*: immediate beta-blockade interrupts the damaging sudden rise in sympathetic tone and protects the heart from overload. It may limit the size of the infarct and reduce risk of arrhythmia but may also precipitate acute heart failure and therefore should not be given at home within the first few hours.)

– for heart failure:
    – frusemide or combination of frusemide with amiloride or of triamterene with a thiazide;
    – if there is no evidence of heart failure, it is best to avoid thiazides because they stimulate the renin – angiotensin system and make the heart work harder (see p.15).
    – for angina: it is a good idea for every patient to have a supply of GTN in case of need even if he has not actually experienced any angina.

– for arrhythmias (see p.238):
    – reconsider admission to hospital;

- beta-blocker unless contra-indicated;
- if beta-blocker contra-indicated (e.g. by heart failure or history of asthma) another agent may be needed but all have side-effects, some of which are serious.

- for emboli:
  - reconsider admission to hospital;
  - anticoagulate: take blood for prothrombin time; then give warfarin 10 mg stat, monitor prothrombin time.

The management of acute myocardial infarction is summarized in Table 4.2F.

Table 4.2F Treatment of acute myocardial infarction

Collapse	Resuscitation
Pain	Diamorphine Cyclizine
Coronary perfusion	Nitrates Aspirin
Bradycardia	Atropine
Tachycardia	Lignocaine
Heart failure	Frusemide Oxygen

The road to recovery

Rehabilitation

This starts at once. Success depends as much on the interest of the doctor and his ability to taylor his advice to the specific needs of the individual patient as on the active and enthusiastic cooperation of the patient and his family. A local course, run specially for the purpose, is a great advantage. Activity should be graded according to how the patient feels and it should be of a kind that the patient chooses and enjoys. Many find it difficult to decide, for themselves, what to do and when; the patient may nag the doctor to lay down rigid rules or, worse, the family may ask the doctor to intervene "Tell him he mustn't do it, Doctor". The doctor should resist: every patient's needs and capabilities are different; each progresses at a different rate; for the rest of his life, the patient is going to have to arrange his own activities, calibrating what he can do against any disability he may have. Rehabilitation is not doing what the doctor tells you, it is learning to make the most of what you can do yourself. The doctor's role in this is to offer guidelines and support; a leaflet may help.

At least 75% of patients can return to work within 3 months of their infarct.

A plan for the patient

At the last home visit or on discharge from hospital, i.e. about 10 days after the infarct, it is helpful to draw up a *rehabilitation plan* with the patient, to cover the next few weeks.

The plan should include the following items plus anything else which the patient wants included:

(1) Principle of graded activity.

(2) Warnings about significant symptoms – and what to report to the doctor:
- urgently;
- at the next convenient opportunity;
- at the next arranged visit.

(3) Provisional date for return to work, if appropriate. This should take into account:
- the severity of the infarct and any subsequent complications;
- the patient's age;
- the type of work: heavy; stressful; dangerous; requiring HGV, PSV or taxi licence;
- the attitude of the employer: would he agree to light work; short hours, at least to start with?
- the home circumstances: happy and peaceful or chaotic and strife-riven?

A firm decision will have to be delayed for several weeks, until the extent of recovery can be assessed.

(4) Drugs

(a) All patients should take:

- A cardio-selective beta-blocker (e.g. metoprolol 50 mg three times a day, unless contra-indicated (heart failure, history of

asthma, severe peripheral vascular disease see Chapter 2.3 p.59). This has been shown to reduce mortality during the next 2 years and is definitely to be recommended in high risk patients. High-risk patients are defined as those with acute myocardial infarction who:
- had chronic angina before the infarct;
- have recurrent pain after the infarct;
- have hypertension;
- have late arrhythmias i.e. ventricular arrhythmias after the first 24 h;
- have had pulmonary oedema;
- have ischaemic changes on ECG in a part of the heart remote from the infarct during an effort test after recovering.
  - Low-risk patients have such a good prognosis anyway that it is less important for them;
    - aspirin: 75–150 mg (1/4 to 1/2 an ordinary tablet) once a day lessens the reinfarction rate by reducing platelet stickiness;
  - GTN supply in case required.

(b) Treatment for complicating conditions: see chapters on heart failure, hypertension, arrhythmias, angina.

(c) The patient must be quite clear what each drug is for, when he should take it, whether there are likely to be any side-effects and about any special instructions.

This is especially important for a drug, such as GTN, the effectiveness of which depends on its being taken for the correct indication (chest pain); in the correct way (sub-lingually); at the correct time (before or at the onset of the pain); and which has a common and potentially, worrying side-effect (headache); and special instructions as to storage and life.

(4) Follow-up appointment:
It is important that the patient has an appointment to see his GP even if he also has one at the hospital.

In hospital outpatients, he is likely to be flustered and ill at ease. He may be seen by a young and inexperienced doctor, whom he has never met before. Even if the technical problems are efficiently handled, not all the necessary ground can possibly be covered. This is the GP's job.

Follow-up appointments should be made at three weeks, at six weeks and then long term.

Follow-up at three weeks

This should be at the surgery unless the patient is too disabled or the journey impossible.

(1) Check:

  – general condition: how does he feel?

  – specific symptoms: chest pain, orthopnoea, paroxysmal nocturnal dyspnoea, breathlessness, palpitations, funny turns or faints, swollen ankles.

  – anxieties?

  – smoking: prognosis depends more on this than on any other factor.

  – drug regime:
      – is it appropriate?
      – is it being adhered to?
      – are there any side-effects?
        (No Brownie points for trying to do without the GTN, if it is needed.)

  – is he coping with graded exercise?

  – is sex OK?
      – if not, is he afraid of it ?
      – does he want to talk about it?
      – it is said that sexual intercourse is equivalent to running up two flights of household stairs, but stairs vary and so do men!

  – does he need help or encouragement in planning his rehabilitation programme?

  – is he making full use of local facilities?

(2) Physical examination:

  · – General condition:
      – does he look good: well, alert, vigorous, good colour?
      – watch for signs of strain, anxiety, depression, fatigue;
      – depression is very common after myocardial infarction.

- Blood pressure: will now be stable and may have reached a new normal for this individual. Treatment given previously for hypertension may now be unnecessary or inappropriate. He may now, for the first time, be found to be hypertensive and need treatment.

- Pulse:
  - tachycardia may indicate compensated heart failure, arrhythmia, anxiety, hyperthyroidism;
  - bradycardia: heart block, too high a dose of beta-blocker, hypothyroidism.

- JVP and liver size: if increased, suggest heart failure.

- Heart sounds: gallop rhythm may suggest heart failure;
  - a new murmur may indicate mitral regurgitation due to heart failure and left ventricular dilatation or possibly a post-infarction ventricular septal defect.

(3)   Investigations: these are necessary only if complications are suspected (e.g. arrhythmia, heart failure, further infarction, ventricular aneurysm) or if the drug regime requires it (e.g. blood urea and electrolytes if taking digoxin, diuretics or ACE inhibitors; thyroid and liver function tests if taking amiodarone).

Follow-up at six weeks

This should repeat all procedures as at three weeks plus:

(1)   ECG even if there are no problems:
  - the S – T segments should now be iso-electric;
  - persistently raised S – T segments suggest the possibility of ventricular aneurysm.

(2)   Blood for lipids and blood sugar.

(3)   Consider referral to a cardiologist for assessment with a view to angioplasty or coronary artery bypass grafting. This should certainly be done if the patient is under 60 years old or having troublesome angina. If he is older and symptom free, then there is no indication for referral.

(4)   Make firm plan for the future:

- is recovery and rehabilitation now complete, both physically and psychologically?
- does he need further help such as physio or gym?
- review lifestyle:
    smoking
    diet
    relationships
    attitudes.
- return to work:
    when?
    should this be the same job?
    short days, short weeks, and light work at first?

The patient should be doing as much during the week or two before returning to work as he expects to be doing when he first returns. Some people find this very difficult and may need to work out a more detailed plan of graded activity, perhaps with a physiotherapist or occupational therapist, if these are available.

Light work and short hours are extremely helpful to ease the person back into work and build up confidence.

Some employers are helpful in this respect and some not.

Follow-up 2 – 4 weeks after returning to work

This is useful to make sure that progress is being maintained and that the patient is coping with the job without symptoms, strain or anxiety. He may need support in not taking on more than he feels he can manage or encouragement to extend himself a bit more.

Long-term follow-up

This should be tailored to the needs of the individual.

A balance has to be struck between the need to allow the person to stop being a patient, and see himself as fully recovered, and the importance of watching out for danger signals and new developments in the progress of the underlying disease process.

A standard plan might be to see the patient every 3 months until the first anniversary of the infarct; every 6 months for the second year and annually thereafter.

(This would be different if the patient were taking any long-term drugs.)

CARDIAC DISEASE

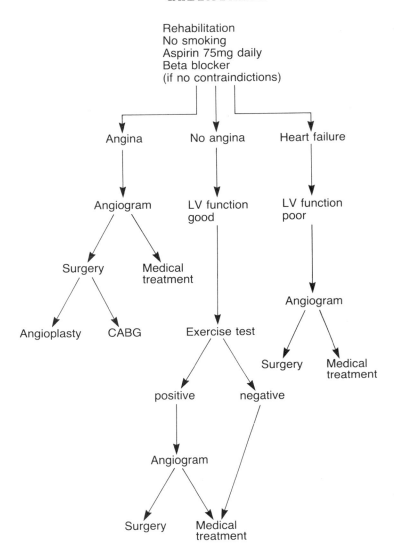

If facilities are limited, age may have to be considered

Figure 4.2Q Later management of myocardial infarction

What to include?
- All procedures as for the check at 3 weeks after infarct.
- Watch for new symptoms; complications; side-effects of drugs.
- Continue support for: active life; non-smoking; healthy diet.

The management of patients following myocardial infarction is summarized in Figure 4.2Q.

What does the future hold?

After 5 years; 47% have died, 40% are disabled and 13% are free from symptoms.

Who benefits from surgery (bypass or angioplasty)?

- Those with proximal mainstem stenosis or three vessel disease live longer.
- Those with angina can expect an improvement in their symptoms.
  See p.171.

What next?

Things are moving very fast in this field.

Some of the most promising new developments are drugs, such as strepto-kinase, anysolated plasminogen streptokinase activator compound (APSAC) and tissue plasminogen activator (TPA), which 'dissolve' thrombus. If given immediately a coronary artery is obstructed and before any muscle death has occurred, these new drugs may actually prevent infarction. It is possible that in the future they may be administered by a GP in the patient's home, by the patient himself or by a relative.

4.3
Heart Failure

INTRODUCTION

In this chapter we examine the different ways in which heart failure manifests itself; what the doctor can expect to find in each situation; the differential diagnoses; and finally the management.

After the usual questions about what it is, what causes it, who gets it and what happens, the effects of heart failure, the symptoms, diagnosis, treatment and long-term care are all discussed separately with respect to:

I.   Acute left heart failure
II. Acute right heart failure
III. Chronic heart failure and congestive heart failure.

WHAT IS IT?

We will use the following definition:

The inability of the heart to maintain an output sufficient for the needs of the body, despite satisfactory venous filling pressure.

This is oversimplified but useful, because it can be applied in a variety of circumstances.

It excludes circulatory failure due to blood loss or anaphylaxis but includes high-output states, where circulatory failure is due to excessive demand more than cardiovascular disease – for example hyperthyroidism or anaemia.

One of the problems with heart failure is that it is not a single condition. In fact, it is not a disease at all but a group of syndromes: each a collection of pathophysiological states. The result of any of them could be described by the definition given above but the differences between them have become important as a result of the tremendous changes in treatment which have become available during recent years.

The way heart failure is managed now makes a significant difference, not only to the quality of life of the individual patient, but to the morbidity and mortality of the condition. Different types of heart failure, with different underlying aetiologies and different consequences, require different treatment.

It is not possible to treat heart failure effectively without making an

200

accurate diagnosis and understanding, as far as possible, the underlying mechanisms.

WHAT CAUSES IT?

The causes (Table 4.3A) may be considered under five broad headings:

(1)   Hyperfunction (excessive demand):
       − sustained (e.g. hypertension);
       − acute (e.g. pulmonary embolism).

(2)   Arrhythmias.

(3)   Loss of contractile tissue.

(4)   Myopathic disorders.

(5)   Pericardial disease.

Table 4.3A Causes of heart failure

HYPERFUNCTION	REDUCED CONTRACTILITY
Hypertension	Chronic ischaemic heart disease
Chronic lung disease	Acute myocardial infarction
Pulmonary embolism	Cardiomyopathy
Valve disease	Acute myocarditis
Hyperthyroidism	Hypothyroidism
REDUCED FILLING	**ARRHYTHMIAS**
Constrictive pericarditis	Bradycardias
Pericardial effusion	Tachycardias

Hyperfunction

Pure left ventricular failure results from conditions which demand increased work of the left ventricle alone. Examples are hypertension and aortic stenosis.

Hyperthyroidism demands increased work of both ventricles and is commonly associated with congestive (biventricular) failure.

Pure right ventricular failure results from long-standing chronic lung disease with raised pulmonary vascular resistance (cor pulmonale) or, rarely, from pulmonary stenosis or primary pulmonary hypertension. Massive pulmonary embolism causes acute right ventricular failure.

Mitral stenosis produces complex effects because although when heart failure develops the symptoms are those of left heart failure, the left ventricle is not under stress. The strain is on the right ventricle, which has to work harder because of increased pulmonary arterial pressure. Therefore, pulmonary oedema and a low left ventricular output, accompanied by severe symptoms, may be followed by the onset of right ventricular failure and improvement in symptoms as the pressure is taken off the lungs.

Loss of contractile tissue

This usually results from myocardial infarction and is most likely to affect the left ventricle so that left ventricular failure predominates. However, both ventricles are often affected, resulting in congestive failure and, rarely, the right ventricle alone fails.

Myopathic disorders

Cardiomyopathies, including those associated with ischaemic heart disease, usually affect both ventricles. However, the left ventricle sustains far higher pressures than the right and is likely to show signs of failure first.

In hypertrophic obstructive cardiomyopathy (HOCM), the addition of left ventricular outflow tract narrowing (aortic sub-valvar stenosis) adds the strain of sustained hyperfunction to the myocardium weakened by myopathy and hastens the onset of left ventricular failure.

The type of heart failure depends on the underlying cause and on the presence of other factors. Very often more than one condition contributes to the overall picture. For instance, hypertensive heart failure is commonly associated with ischaemic heart disease.

Acute heart failure may be precipitated by a factor quite distinct from the underlying cause. For instance, a patient with angina may develop heart failure when an already compromised myocardium is further depressed by a beta-blocker. Heart failure may be triggered by a chest infection, by a small myocardial infarct or by the sudden onset of atrial fibrillation, none of which would have caused heart failure on their own. It is important to recognise these precipitating causes as they may be more amenable to treatment than the underlying disease.

Table 4.3B Precipitating causes of heart failure

Myocardial infarction
Arrhythmias
Acute infections
Hyperthyroidism
Anaemia
Subacute bacterial endocarditis
Drugs: beta-blockers, NSAIDS, medicines with high sodium content (e.g. antacids)
Poor compliance with treatment for heart failure or hypertension

Who suffers heart failure?

Heart failure occurs only as a result of underlying disease. Therefore, those who develop heart failure are among those who suffer from the underlying diseases. Whatever the main pathology, the risk of heart failure is worse for those whose cardiac function is adversely influenced by other factors: smoking, hypertension, hyperlipidaemia, diabetes.

WHAT HAPPENS?

The natural history of heart failure has been obscured by the effectiveness and availability of modern treatment. Any observations have to be interpreted with this in mind. The mortality of severe heart failure is 50% in a year. Of these, half suffer sudden cardiac death (SCD). The likelihood of SCD is proportional to the degree of ventricular dilatation. This is partly because ventricular dilatation is arrhythmogenic.

Symptoms are unreliable indicators of the severity of the condition and of prognosis. Here, for instance, is a comparison of two patients (with thanks to Dr Celia Oakley).

Patient 1 has left ventricular failure with pulmonary oedema and severe symptoms.
His left ventricle is not dilated.
He has:
  – an ejection fraction of 40% (slightly reduced);
  – a stroke volume of 60 ml (slightly reduced);
  – an LV end diastolic pressure of 30 mm (severely raised).
His prognosis is quite good.

Patient 2 has left ventricular failure with no symptoms at rest.
His left ventricle is dilated.

He has:
- an ejection fraction of 20% (severely reduced);
- a stroke volume of 100 ml (normal);
- an LV end diastolic pressure of 15 mm (moderately raised).

His prognosis is very poor.

The first patient has the more efficient heart. The left ventricle pumps out 40% of its total volume at every beat (normal is only about 60%). The symptoms are due to the fact that the end diastolic pressure is raised so high that pulmonary oedema has developed. This is because the end diastolic pressure is the same as the pressure in the left atrium and therefore the same as that in the pulmonary veins and in the lungs themselves. The myocardium is in better shape than that of Patient 2 and, with appropriate treatment, will last longer.

The second patient can manage an ejection fraction of only 20%. However, because of his dilated ventricle, this results in a normal stroke volume. The end diastolic pressure is raised but not enough to cause pulmonary oedema. The myocardium is in very poor condition, the Frank – Starling mechanism is lost and will soon give up altogether, even if he does not suffer SCD. No treatment is going to help very much.

Compensatory mechanisms

The main homeostatic mechanisms in the cardiovascular system are designed to maintain a normal cardiac output in terms of pressure and volume. Whenever the cardiac output falls, the body behaves as if the person were bleeding and does all it can to maintain the blood pressure and replace the lost volume.

The sympathetic nervous system is stimulated by a fall in blood pressure detected by baroceptors in the aorta and carotid sinuses. The results of this are peripheral vasoconstriction, increased myocardial contractility and increased heart rate.

The renin – angiotensin – aldosterone system is stimulated by the fall in renal perfusion. The results of this are peripheral vasoconstriction and increased plasma volume due to salt and water retention.

If the fall in cardiac output is, in fact, due to bleeding, the mechanisms are most effective and produce an increase in blood pressure and in circulating volume to normal levels. This is possible, partly because the heart is normal and can respond to the extra demand by working harder, but also because the increase in plasma volume only restores normal levels and is not associated with a pathological rise in ventricular filling pressure.

If the fall in cardiac output is due to heart failure, the increase in peripheral resistance and circulating blood volume to higher than normal levels, increase the amount of work, further overloading the already failing ventricle. The already raised ventricular filling pressure is increased still further.

In a healthy myocardium, the Frank–Starling mechanism ensures that output is increased when filling pressure rises. The heart works harder and its oxygen consumption increases. In heart failure, the ability to do this is reduced. On the left side, this exacerbates any existing pulmonary oedema. On the right, peripheral oedema is increased.

Figure 4.3A illustrates the mechanisms.

Atrial natriuretic peptide

Serum levels of this substance (or group of substances) are raised in heart failure, possibly as a direct result of raised intra-atrial pressure. It acts as a vasodilator, especially on renal arterioles and as a mild potassium-sparing diuretic. It does this partly by increasing glomerular filtration rate, reducing the activation of the renin–angiotensin–aldosterone system, and partly by inhibiting aldosterone. Its effects are, to a great extent, overshadowed by the vasoconstrictor mechanisms outlined above but it may have therapeutic implications when it is better understood.

Knowledge of the way the homeostatic mechanisms work has been used to develop drugs for the treatment of heart failure. For instance, spironolactone blocks the action of aldosterone and therefore reduces retention of salt and water. ACE inhibitors, acting farther back in the chain, block the formation of angiotensin II from angiotensin I and also reduce the production of aldosterone. The overall effects of these drugs is extremely complex but it is necessary to have some idea of how and where they act if they are to be used intelligently.

WHAT EFFECT DOES HEART FAILURE HAVE?

The effects of heart failure are dramatically different depending on:
>   the underlying cause
>   which chamber of the heart is primarily affected
>   whether the condition is acute or chronic
>   whether the patient is taking cardiac drugs.

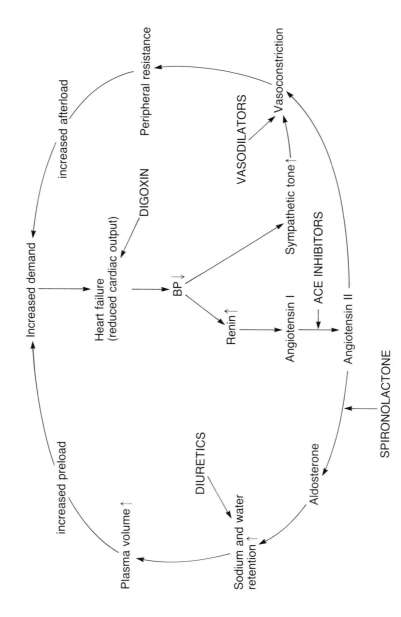

Figure 4.3A Mechanisms in heart failure and points at which drugs act

I.   Acute left heart failure

Now that untreated severe mitral stenosis is uncommon, this is most likely to be left ventricular failure (LVF) due to acute myocardial infarction. The clinical picture is usually complicated by pain, fear and shock, but silent infarction, causing acute LVF, is also common.

Uncomplicated acute LVF has two areas of effect: the lungs and the systemic output.

The lungs

(1)   The left ventricle is suddenly unable to pump onwards the blood reaching it from the lungs.

(2)   The right ventricle continues to pump normally.

(3)   The left atrial pressure rises and the lungs become waterlogged: pulmonary oedema.

This is sometimes called backward failure.

The patient is severely breathless. He finds that he is more comfortable sitting up. Attempts to get him to lie down increase his distress. This is because the venous return to the right heart is reduced in the upright posture, which reduces right ventricular output and the blood flow to the lungs.

Vasodilators such as nitrates have a beneficial effect similar to the upright posture, pooling blood in the lower limbs and reducing venous return to the heart.

Systemic output

(1)   The output of the left ventricle is reduced.

(2)   The blood pressure falls.

(3)   The patient may feel dizzy, lose consciousness, and develop Cheyne–Stokes breathing.

This is sometimes called forward failure.

The changes described so far are the immediate haemodynamic changes which result from failure of the left ventricular pump.

The remaining acute changes are those resulting from the activation of the homeostatic mechanisms described previously. These cause tachycardia, peripheral vasoconstriction (with pallor), sweating, oliguria, thirst.

Why is LVF so often missed?

Left ventricular failure is commonly acute but intermittent and can then present diagnostic problems for the doctor. It is not present when the patient is seen. The diagnosis is made entirely on the history. This will be discussed later but an understanding of the underlying mechanisms helps to avoid missing the diagnosis.

The left ventricle may be perfectly capable of maintaining an adequate output when the patient is upright, at rest or pottering gently. It fails only when demand is increased, as in exercise, or when the right ventricular output increases, as it does on lying down. Thus the patient gives a history of cough and breathlessness on exertion, on lying down (orthopnoea), or during the night (paroxysmal nocturnal dyspnoea), but may have no abnormal physical signs.

CAMEO

Mrs Maureen Brooks, aged 64, asked the doctor to call as she had become breathless and could not take her dog for a walk. She had a cough and wheezy chest which was worse at night, when she had to sit up to get her breath.

The doctor discovered that she had had an episode of chest pain a week previously which she ascribed to indigestion.

On examination she was breathless, pulse regular, 100/min, BP 120/80, JVP normal, no oedema, heart sounds I and II normal with third sound audible at the apex.

A diagnosis of left ventricular failure was made and she was treated with frusemide 40 mg daily reducing to 20 mg daily after one week. She was able to stop it altogether six weeks later.

An ECG confirmed a recent myocardial infarct.

II. Acute right heart failure

This may be due to acute myocardial infarction, involving the right ventricle, or to massive pulmonary embolism. As with acute left heart failure, the picture may be confused by pain, fear and shock. The right ventricle is suddenly unable to pump onward the blood reaching it from the periphery. Insufficient blood reaches the left ventricle for the needs of the body. The left ventricular output falls. The systemic blood pressure falls. The systemic venous pressure (observed as JVP) is raised.

The effects of this are that the patient feels faint, especially if made to sit up. He is more comfortable lying down as this increases the right ventricular filling pressure and increases right ventricular output (Frank–Starling mechanism). He is not breathless unless the underlying cause is pulmonary embolism. If he has had a pulmonary embolus, he is breathless but is not made worse by lying down. This is because his breathlessness is not due to raised pulmonary venous pressure: he does not have pulmonary oedema.

His main problem is reduced right ventricular output. Any reduction in right ventricular filling pressure, such as might result from sitting up, reduces the right ventricular output even further and aggravates the problem.

Diuretics and vasodilators, which cause peripheral venodilatation, reduce the systemic venous pressure. This reduces the right ventricular filling pressure. Right ventricular output is further reduced, and this can have disastrous effects.

A patient with acute LVF due to myocardial infarction and another with acute RVF due to pulmonary embolism may, at first glance, appear similar. Both have chest pain, breathlessness and a reduced cardiac output, with tachycardia and possibly hypotension. It is of the utmost importance to distinguish between them as treatment appropriate for one could kill the other.

III.   Chronic heart failure

In all forms of chronic heart failure, compensatory mechanisms dominate the picture.

Chronic left heart failure

This is unusual nowadays because of modern management of the underlying causes, especially mitral stenosis, aortic valve disease and hypertension.

The main compensatory mechanisms are those affecting the lungs. These are:

(1)   pulmonary arteriolar constriction, which reduces flow into the capillaries and increases pulmonary arterial pressure;

(2)   right ventricular failure resulting from increased pulmonary vascular resistance, partly due to (1) above;

(3)   increased pulmonary lymphatic flow, which removes some of the excess fluid from the lungs.

Chronic right heart failure

This is usually due to long-standing chronic lung disease, which increases the stiffness of the lungs and the resistance to flow of blood through them. It is then called cor pulmonale.

It is characterised by the effects of back pressure and of hypervolaemia due to fluid retention: raised RV filling pressure (JVP), enlarged liver, peripheral (dependent) oedema, ascites and cardiac cirrhosis with jaundice.

Chronic congestive (biventricular) heart failure

This has characteristics of both left and right heart failure but an important difference is that the failure of the right ventricle protects the lungs from the worst effects of left heart failure.

There is little or no pulmonary oedema unless some acute event, such as a myocardial infarct, intervenes.

The important elements of left heart failure are those which reduce output (forward failure). This is responsible for limiting exercise and for activating the renin – angiotensin – aldosterone system. Nocturia may occur due to increased production of antidiuretic hormone (ADH).

The contributions of the failure of the right ventricle to this syndrome are the same as those listed above for chronic right heart failure.

WHAT DO YOU FIND?

As a rule, the diagnosis of left heart failure is made on the strength of the history and symptoms; that of right heart failure on the physical findings and congestive heart failure or a combination of the two.

I. Acute left heart failure

Left heart failure (LHF) is usually acute but it may be repeated or prolonged, especially if not recognised or inadequately treated. It is often intermittent so that the patient has no complaints when visiting the doctor.

The patient often interprets the symptoms for the doctor: 'I am chesty again doctor; bronchitis, you know. I think I need some of your antibiotics.'

This sort of complaint should always put the doctor on the alert. If the patient is young, it is likely to be bronchial asthma; if older, cardiac asthma (LHF).

Simple chest infections are not particularly common.

Hallmarks of LHF

(1)   breathlessness:
        – on exertion (exertional dyspnoea);
        – on lying down (orthopnoea);
        – during the night (paroxysmal nocturnal dyspnoea, PND);
        – accompanied by cough, sometimes with pink, frothy sputum forces
          patient to stop, get out of bed, stand or sit.

(2)   fatigue and weakness.

(3)   cerebral symptoms: dizziness, confusion, Cheyne–Stokes respiration.

(4)   pulmonary venous congestion or frank pulmonary oedema on chest
        X-ray.

There are likely to be symptoms or signs of the underlying cause, such as
ischaemic heart disease or hypertension and also of an immediate
precipitating factor, such as atrial fibrillation.

Therefore, a careful history and examination are important, even if the
diagnosis of the LHF itself is beyond doubt.

An ECG and chest X-ray are necessary to complete the diagnosis.

If the patient is seen during a continuing attack of acute LHF, there will
be signs of:
        – pulmonary oedema: râles throughout both lung fields (basal râles are
          universal, especially in the elderly and rarely of any significance);
        – bronchospasm (hence the term 'cardiac asthma'): disappears after a
          short time;
        – reduced LV output: pallor, hypotension;
        – sympathetic hyperactivity:
                tachycardia,
                peripheral vasoconstriction (pallor, cold extremities)
                sweating
                dry mouth
                hypertension;
        – gallop rhythm.

The blood pressure is an unreliable sign. It may be:
        – low because the left ventricle is so weak that it cannot sustain a higher
          level;
        – low because the patient is taking hypotensive drugs: nitrates and
          beta-blockers are likely culprits;
        – normal because the patient is usually hypertensive but the left
          ventricle cannot keep up its usual level (decapitated hypertension);

211

- high because the patient is hypertensive;
- high as a result of sympathetic stimulation increasing myocardial contractility and peripheral vasoconstriction.

A low blood pressure, or decapitated hypertension, which cannot be explained by drugs is a bad prognostic sign, suggesting a severely damaged myocardium.

II.   Acute right heart failure

Acute right heart failure (RHF) can be due to massive pulmonary embolism or acute myocardial infarction. In both, chest pain may predominate. Breathlessness is the main feature in pulmonary embolism. Right heart failure results in two groups of physical findings:

(1)   Those due to reduced cardiac output:
- poor peripheral perfusion;
- hypotension (but see above about BP in LVF);
- results of sympathetic stimulation (see under LVF);
- results of reduced renal perfusion.

(2)   Those due to back pressure:
- raised JVP;
- large, tender liver;
- peripheral (dependent) oedema (sacral or ankle);
- ascites.

Oedema and ascites may not be immediately apparent but develop within a few hours, being made worse by the salt and water retention and hypervolaemia, which are caused by the activation of the renin–angiotensin–aldosterone system.

III.   Chronic and congestive heart failure

Chronic right heart failure

This affects people with long-standing chronic lung disease and is usually expected. The main problem arises from the tendency of doctors to anticipate the diagnosis and treat peripheral oedema which is in fact due to another cause, such as immobility, as if it were heart failure. The result is that many people are given diuretics unnecessarily and with undesirable results.

The findings in cor pulmonale are:

(1)   Those due to back pressure from the failing right ventricle (backward failure):
- raised JVP;
- enlarged liver, cirrhosis, jaundice;
- peripheral (dependent) oedema;
- ascites.

(2)   Those due to reduced cardiac output (forward failure):
- cold extremities;
- confusion, dizziness;
- fatigue;
- hypervolaemia (from activation of renin system).

(3)   Those due to the underlying lung disease:
- cough;
- breathlessness;
- malaise/ fatigue.

Congestive heart failure

The clinical picture is dominated by the underlying disease and the immediate precipitating factor.

A typical situation might be someone who has a history of ischaemic heart disease with a myocardial infarct or angina in the past. Over a few days, he develops:

palpitations	increased fatigue
breathlessness	ankle oedema
increased angina	mild confusion.

He is found to have:
- a fast, irregular pulse (ECG confirms atrial fibrillation);
- raised JVP;
- an enlarged heart;
- enlarged, tender liver;
- oedema of feet and ankles;
- cold extremities.

The precipitating factor is the onset of atrial fibrillation: ventricular filling time is reduced by the tachycardia and myocardial contractility, reduced by the ischaemic heart disease, cannot increase enough to compensate.

The underlying pathology is ischaemic heart disease.

The raised jugular venous pressure, hepatomegaly and oedema are due to back pressure from the failing right ventricle.

The fatigue, confusion and cold extremities are due to reduced peripheral perfusion and this also contributes to the oedema by causing hypervolaemia via the renin system.

The fall in output stimulates the sympathetic system. This increases heart rate and thus myocardial oxygen demands, aggravates the angina and makes the cold extremities worse by vasoconstriction.

The breathlessness is due to raised pulmonary venous pressure caused by failure of the left ventricle.

WHAT ELSE MIGHT IT BE?

Acute left heart failure

There are two main areas of difficulty:

(1)   Acute left heart failure due to acute myocardial infarction may be confused with right heart failure due to massive pulmonary embolism.

Both conditions may be characterised by severe central chest pain, devastating breathlessness and a low cardiac output.

The most useful clinical distinguishing feature is the effect of position on the patient's symptoms.

A patient with left heart failure vigorously resists lying down and becomes more breathless if made to do so.

A patient with acute right heart failure does not object to lying down and may feel better if he does so.

(2)   Acute bronchial asthma: even if the patient is seen during the attack, it may be impossible to distinguish acute LHF from acute bronchial asthma without a chest X-ray.

However, there may be some clues.

Bronchial asthma

–   The patient is younger (but watch out for late-onset asthma).

–   History of:
     wheezy attacks (unlike LHF)
     atopy; eczema, allergy
     childhood asthma

214

exercise asthma
nocturnal asthma, not improved by getting up.

- Recent likely trigger: URTI, emotional upset (but these can trigger LHF too).

- Bronchospasm persists for more than an hour.

- Peak flow rate is persistently low.

- Breathlessness relieved by inhaled beta-agonist (e.g. salbutamol) but wheeze due to *early* acute LHF is also relieved by inhaled beta-agonists.

Cardiac asthma (LHF)

- The patient is older.

- There is known underlying disease e.g. hypertension, ischaemic heart disease.

- There are multiple IHD risk factors: smoking, obesity, diabetes, hypertension, family history of IHD.

- Recent history is typical of intermittent LHF or suggestive of ischaemic heart disease (e.g. angina, acute MI).

- Bronchospasm is shortlived but breathlessness persists.

- Precipitating cause, such as sudden onset of arrhythmia.

- Relief given by i.v. frusemide.

- ECG signs of LV strain, MI or ischaemia.

Beta-blockers can confuse matters, since they can precipitate either. They also limit the heart rate response in both conditions. Anyone who develops 'bronchitis' soon after starting a beta-blocker must be considered as a candidate for both bronchial and cardiac asthma.

If in doubt, do not give opiates (dangerous in bronchial asthma) nor systemic steroids (not helpful in acute LHF).

If it is impossible to obtain a chest X-ray, it is reasonable, in an emergency, to give both a loop diuretic (frusemide) and an inhaled beta-agonist (salbutamol) together with i.v. aminophylline. For management, see p.216.

II.   Right heart failure

Patients with severe, chronic lung disease are often inactive.

They develop ankle oedema due to stasis. On its own, this is not enough to make a diagnosis of cor pulmonale.

III.   Congestive heart failure

There is a temptation to label any elderly person, with oedema of the ankles, as suffering from congestive heart failure.

Peripheral oedema is very common. It affects women of all ages and elderly people of both sexes, especially in hot weather or when sitting about a lot. Journeys by air are particularly likely to cause it. Many people return from holiday with swollen feet. They do not have heart failure and should not be given diuretics.

Rarely, renal disease, giving rise to oedema, causes confusion. The cardinal rule is:

IF OEDEMA IS DUE TO HEART FAILURE,
THE JUGULAR VENOUS PRESSURE IS RAISED

WHAT DO YOU DO?

I.   Acute left heart failure

Acute left heart failure (pulmonary oedema) is a medical emergency. An attack may resolve spontaneously, for instance if the patient stops the activity which precipitated it, or even if he simply sits up in bed – but it may be fatal and there is no way of knowing, when the telephone call comes at 4 a.m., which way it will end.

Even if this attack resolves spontaneously, if appropriate treatment is not given, it will recur. It is one of the few situations where medication makes a significant difference to the outcome.

The aims of treatment

(1)   To reduce the venous return to the heart.

(2)   To effect a diuresis.

(3)   To identify the underlying disease and precipitating cause and treat them, if possible.

(4)   To prevent further attacks.

        Action:
        – sit the patient up with legs down.
        – give:
            – a rapidly acting nitrate (e.g. sublingual GTN);
            – frusemide: 40 mg i.v. slowly;
            – diamorphine 5 mg with cyclizine 25 mg i.v. slowly;
            – oxygen, intermittently, for short periods.
        – if the patient does not improve very rapidly:
            – give aminophylline 250 – 500 mg i.v. slowly;
            – a light tourniquet (e.g. a sphygmomanometer cuff), inflated to
              about 50 mmHg, around each thigh, may reduce the venous
              return enough to allow the pulmonary oedema to resolve;
            – admit to hospital.
            (If the patient is already taking aminophylline, do not give the
            intravenous dose.)
        – identify and treat the underlying cause and precipitating factor.
          These may be known or immediately obvious. Arrhythmias and
          acute myocardial infarction associated with pulmonary oedema are
          usually best admitted hospital. It may be better to keep some
          patients at home. This can only be decided by the doctor on the
          spot.

If the patient stays at home, he will need:
        – full clinical assessment;
        – an ECG to check for:
            – acute myocardial infarction,
            – arrhythmias;
        – blood for cardiac enzymes;
        – to be seen later the same day and reassessed;
        – a long-term treatment plan to prevent further attacks, see below.
          This will include a diuretic and treatment for any other conditions
          (e.g. digoxin for atrial fibrillation; hypotensive drugs for hyper-
          tension).

Intermittent attacks

The diagnosis of LHF is often made between attacks (see p.208). It is
important to identify and treat these promptly as the next attack may be fatal.
The short-term aims are:
(1)   To confirm the diagnosis.
(2)   To treat the heart failure with a diuretic.

(3)   To identify the underlying cause and any precipitating factors.
(4)   To treat these other conditions.

For long-term management of left heart failure, see below.

II.   Chronic right heart failure due to cor pulmonale

Whilst it is useful to recognise the development of right heart failure in a patient with chronic lung disease, the lung disease remains the main problem.

The best treatment consists of giving the smallest dose of a potassium-sparing diuretic which will reduce the jugular venous pressure to near normal and paying meticulous attention to the lung disease.

It may not be possible to remove all the oedema without giving an overdose of diuretic and producing undesirable side-effects due to electrolyte disturbance and reduced cardiac output. These include fatigue, dizzyness, confusion and dehydration and can make the patient very miserable.

III.   Congestive heart failure

It must be remembered that this is not itself a diagnosis. There must be an underlying disease, maybe more than one. There may be precipitating factors. The condition cannot be satisfactorily treated until a complete set of diagnoses has been made.

The treatment will consist of:
– initial diuretics with possible addition of ACE inhibitor later;
– appropriate treatment of other conditions;
– long-term follow-up (see below).

LONG-TERM MANAGEMENT OF HEART FAILURE

The long-term aims

(1)   To prevent further attacks of left heart failure.
(2)   To minimise disability in all patients.

The details of management

These will vary enormously depending on:
– the age, frailty and wishes of the patient;
– the nature and severity of the underlying disease;

- the response to treatment;
- the presence of coexisting disease or disability;
- the facilities available in the area.

General guidelines

Only general guidelines can be given here:

- Most patients will need to take diuretics for the rest of their lives.

- If the precipitating factor is one which can be completely controlled, e.g. atrial fibrillation, then it may be possible to stop the diuretic or substitute a milder one.

- Diuretics activate the renin–angiotensin system, increasing peripheral resistance. This, combined with the reduction in plasma volume which they cause, further reduces cardiac output.

- Therefore, if a long-term diuretic is needed, it should be the smallest effective dose of a potassium-sparing one or combination (e.g. frusemide and amiloride). If a dose of more than 40 mg frusemide daily is needed, it is likely that the patient will benefit from the cautious addition of an ACE inhibitor. If this is done, then the potassium-sparing diuretic should be omitted.

- Regular checks of blood urea and electrolytes are necessary.

- Hyperkalaemia causes muscular weakness and arrhythmias.
    - It can be caused by potassium-sparing diuretics, especially if the patient takes potassium supplements with them. It is more likely to occur if the blood urea is raised.
    - The ECG shows tall, spiky T waves (Figure 4.3B).

- Hypokalaemia causes muscular weakness, arrhythmias and constipation. It makes arrhythmias, due to digoxin, more likely.
    - The ECG shows flat T waves and depressed S–T segments.

- Specific enquiry should be made for exertional dyspnoea, orthopnoea and paroxysmal nocturnal dyspnoea.

- If the symptoms are not controlled, the addition of a peripheral vasodilator, such as a long-acting nitrate, ACE inhibitor or calcium-channel blocker, may help. ACE inhibitors can cause profound hypo-

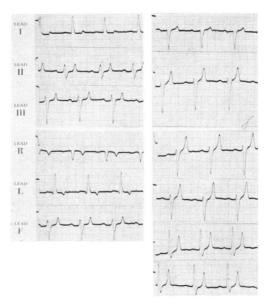

Figure 4.3B ECG in hyperkalaemia

tension in heart failure and care is needed, see p.72. At this stage, referral to a consultant may be useful.

Who do you refer to hospital?

Emergency

Left heart failure which:
- fails to respond to treatment;
- is associated with a condition which itself requires admission (e.g. acute myocardial infarction or arrhythmia).

Outpatient clinic

Patients:
- in whom the diagnosis is not clear;
- who may need further investigation (e.g. possible valve disease or assessment of ischaemic heart disease);
- who fail to respond to treatment either of the failure or of the underlying condition.

4.4
Essential Hypertension

WHAT IS IT?

Essential hypertension describes the finding of systemic blood pressure, above normal, for which no cause can be found.

Like all other physiological measurements, the normal blood pressure represents a range. It is a variable and repeated measurements are needed to establish a true picture in any individual.

A reasonable, if rough, working definition of the upper limit of normal is:

Systolic: 100 + age;

Diastolic: 90 for people under 50
100 for people 50 – 70
110 for people over 70.

For the purposes of this chapter, we are going to use the figures in Table 4.4A to define hypertension.

Table 4.4A Hypertension

	Systolic	Diastolic (5th phase)		
		< 50 years	*50 – 70 years*	*> 70 years*
Mild	> 100 + age	90 – 100	100 – 110	110 – 120
Moderate	> 120 + age	100 – 110	110 – 120	120 – 130
Severe	> 130 + age	> 110	> 120	> 130

These are arbitary figures. They do not form part of any recognisable set of generally accepted criteria: there are none. They serve as a baseline only: a set of default figures to fall back on if needed.

Malignant hypertension is defined as hypertension causing papilloedema.

The diagnosis of hypertension is based on a minimum of three readings taken on different days and at different times.

Even if the first reading is extremely high and it is obvious that the patient has hypertension, at least three readings, at well spaced intervals, are needed to establish the severity of the condition and a baseline before starting treatment.

CAMEO

Ronald Christie is 42, a salesman, with numerous domestic and financial problems. He came to the surgery late one afternoon feeling exhausted and harrassed. His blood pressure was 238/134, taken twice. He had no other symptoms and no papilloedema or proteinurea. His ECG was normal. He was advised to take some time off work and to return to the surgery in a few days. Three days later, he was feeling better and his blood pressure was 215/120. Further readings taken at weekly intervals were 190/118 and 194/112.

WHO HAS HYPERTENSION?

Of the adult population:
    20% have mild hypertension;
    15% have moderate hypertension;
    5% have severe hypertension.

It is more likely to affect those with a family history of hypertension in a close relative: parent or sibling.

A GP with a list of 2000 patients can expect to have a total of 800 patients with hypertension. Half of these will have mild hypertension and most will be over 40 years old. The rule of halves is a useful guide.

The rule of halves

Of 800 people with hypertension:
    ½ (400) are known;
    ½ of these (200) are treated;
    ½ of these (100) are well-controlled.

WHAT CAUSES IT?

There have been a number of theories but none is completely satisfactory. Part of the difficulty lies in sorting out which findings, commonly associated with hypertension, are the result of the raised blood pressure, which are associated effects of the underlying cause and which are part of the causal process itself.

There are number of factors which are known to be important in the prognosis for patients with hypertension and which may form part of the causal mechanisms, at least in some people. These include all those risk factors which are significant for coronary heart disease (see p.311):

Male sex	Diabetes
Obesity	Hyperlipidaemia
Alcohol consumption	Atheroma
Salt intake	Left ventricular hypertrophy
Smoking	Oral contraceptive use
Stress	Family history.

The importance of these factors varies from one individual to another.

Higher readings of blood pressure are obtained using a normal size cuff on a very fat patient but even allowing for this, obesity is clearly significant. If an obese hypertensive patient loses weight, the blood pressure is likely to fall: about 5 mmHg for every 5 kg weight.

Alcohol abuse seems to be an important aetiological factor in some patients. Since it is impossible to tell which they are, it is sensible to advise all hypertensives to drink moderately, if at all.

Similarly, some hypertensives can reduce their blood pressure by changing to a low-salt diet. It does not work for all but it is presumably an integral part of the mechanism in those for whom it does.

Hypertension affects non-smokers as well as smokers, but it makes a significant difference to the outcome as well as to the effectiveness of treatment. It is not clear whether it is itself a causative factor.

Stress has the effect of raising the blood pressure in normal people for short periods. It is part of the physiological fight/flight defence mechanism. It has been postulated that, in people who are subject to frequent or continuous stress, the baroreceptors are reset at a higher level. This would have the effect of making their 'normal' blood pressure pathologically high with all the resultant effects.

The combination of diabetes and hypertension is common and is bad news prognostically. The cause and effect equation is, again, impossible to disentangle. Diabetes is associated with obesity, so is hypertension; diabetes is associated with atheroma, so is hypertension; diabetes is associated with renal disease, so is hypertension. It is these interwoven relationships which make the combination of the two conditions so dangerous.

It is unlikely that atheroma is a direct cause of hypertension but it is certain that, when the two conditions coexist, the risks are greatly increased.

Hypertension runs in families and most patients can think of a relative with it. If both parents have hypertension, half their children will be affected. If one parent is affected, the risk is one in four.

Two of the main homeostatic mechanisms in the body have the effect of increasing the blood pressure under physiological conditions. These are:

(1) The sympathetic nervous system, acting in response to:
  – a reduction in blood pressure detected by the baroreceptors in the aortic arch and carotid bodies;
  – stress (e.g. pain or fear);
  – exercise;
  The increase in blood pressure results from selective increase in peripheral arteriolar constriction and also an increase in contractility of the myocardium.

(2) The renin–angiotensin system, stimulated by reduced renal blood flow. Angiotensin II is a powerful vasopressor, causing peripheral vasoconstriction. It also causes increased secretion of aldosterone resulting in sodium and fluid retention.

The effects of these mechanisms is normally short term, lasting only a matter of hours. There is no evidence that they cause pathological hypertension.

The ability of the kidneys to excrete sodium is impaired in at least some people with hypertension. Some patients with hypertension have raised renin levels but others do not.

The aetiology of essential hypertension is multifactorial.

HOW DOES HYPERTENSION INTERFERE WITH THE NORMAL FUNCTION OF THE CARDIOVASCULAR SYSTEM?

This is a question which is impossible to answer completely until more is known about the underlying causes of the condition.

For instance, hypertension is associated with a high level of peripheral arteriolar tone. This could be a cause of the high pressure but it is also what would be expected to result from a rise in pressure (see Chapter 1.2).

Increased renal perfusion, associated with hypertension, causes loss of sodium and water and this would be expected to stimulate the renin–angiotensin system. It is not clear whether increased activity in this system is a cause or a result of hypertension.

It is likely that there is, at least to some extent, a vicious circle, in which all or some of the normal homeostatic mechanisms (see Figure 1.3L, p.21) trigger each other to maintain a pathologically high level of blood pressure, at which the baroreceptors are reset.

There is little doubt that the left ventricular hypertrophy of hypertension is a direct result of the extra work the heart has to do to maintain the higher outflow pressure but even this may not be as simple as it seems (see below).

WHAT DOES IT DO?

Hypertension has effects on the heart itself and on the peripheral or target organs: especially the aorta, brain and kidneys.

The main effect on the heart is to cause left ventricular hypertrophy. This is similar to the hypertrophy occurring in any muscle which is used excessively but it is an inconsistent process and the degree of hypertrophy in different individuals does not match the degree of hypertension nor the length of time it has been operating. It appears that, in some people, hypertension may trigger a sort of hypertrophic cardiomyopathy which results in hypertrophy out of all proportion to the levels of blood pressure recorded.

The hypertrophied muscle requires an increased blood supply. If this is not available because of ischaemic heart disease, then angina, myocardial infarction and heart failure, due to ischaemic damage (fibrosis), are likely.

The effects of long-standing hypertension on large to medium-sized arteries are thickening of the vessel wall and increased formation of atheroma. In the coronary arteries, this makes thrombosis and occlusion more likely.

Degeneration of the intimal layers of the aorta is a normal part of ageing. If the blood pressure is raised, in the presence of damaged intima, the likelihood of dissection of the aorta is greatly increased.

The aorta becomes dilated during prolonged hypertension.

The effect of hypertension on the brain can be insidious or cataclysmic. It can cause gradual, progressive deterioration of function, apparently due to the direct effect of the high pressure on the brain. It can be associated with sudden cerebral haemorrhage or thrombosis of a small artery, causing infarction.

Very severe hypertension can cause hypertensive encephalopathy, when the intracranial pressure rises and the patient loses consciousness. Death follows rapidly unless prompt treatment is given.

Hypertension can cause renal damage with proteinuria, uraemia and peripheral oedema. Treatment of the hypertension improves renal function but it is important to exclude underlying primary renal disease.

WHAT HAPPENS?

People with hypertension are more likely to suffer:

Cerebrovascular accident	Angina
Heart failure	Myocardial infarction
Renal failure	Dissection of the aorta.

The higher the blood pressure, the more likely are these complications.

CAMEO

Betty Young is 58 and attends the surgery every 6 months for a blood pressure check. When she was 42, she had a CVA and right hemiplegia while taking an oral contraceptive. Her blood pressure at the time was 178/115. She stopped the pill and was treated with hypotensive drugs. She made a reasonably good recovery but has not worked since and still walks with a limp. Recently, her hypotensive drugs were tailed off and she has remained normotensive without them.

WHY TREAT HYPERTENSION?

Reduction of blood pressure, in anyone with moderate or severe hypertension, reduces the incidence of stroke, heart failure, renal failure and dissection of the aorta. The effect on the risk of myocardial infarction is not so clear-cut.

Hypertension is one of the major risk factors for ischaemic heart disease. The higher the blood pressure, the greater the risk of myocardial infarction. However, it has not yet been possible to prove that drug treatment of hypertension reduces this. This may be because some of the drugs used in trials have themselves introduced a risk, which has obscured any statistical benefit. If this is the case, then new drugs may in the future be found to be effective. Another factor is that the trials of hypotensive treatment, so far reported, have been relatively short. It is probable that a longer period of treatment is necessary before benefit can be demonstrated statistically.

Although mild hypertension reduces life expectancy, the advantages of drug treatment are still being debated. Here is a summary of current thinking:

(1)   Anyone with a diastolic pressure over 100 mmHg persisting for more than 3 months despite non-drug treatment, is likely to benefit from treatment and should be offered a trial of hypotensive drugs.

(2)   Anyone with target organ damage (e.g. LVH, LVF, retinal changes, proteinuria, CVA) should be treated with drugs.

(3)   Enthusiasm for treatment should be greatest in men and in those with other risk factors (see above). Older patients (up to 80 years) should be treated as energetically as anyone else.

(4)   Women with mild hypertension have a very low incidence of complications.

(5)   It is possible that the use of thiazide diuretics in women with mild hypertension may actually increase mortality from coronary heart disease and they are best avoided in this group although, if they smoke, the incidence of stroke is reduced.

(6)   Women with mild hypertension do well on beta-blockers.

(7)   The incidence of stroke in smokers is reduced by thiazide diuretics.

(8)   Propranolol does not improve the outlook for smokers.

(9)   Drug treatment of mild hypertension has not been shown to reduce the incidence of coronary heart disease.

No benefit, in terms of ischaemic heart disease, accrues from having a very low blood pressure, possibly because coronary perfusion, which relies on diastolic pressure, is reduced.

It has been found that reducing diastolic pressure below 80 mmHg is associated with an increased incidence of myocardial infarction. Care should be taken to avoid this.

WHAT DO YOU FIND?

Uncomplicated benign essential hypertension is symptomless.

It is usually diagnosed when the blood pressure is taken as part of a routine examination, for instance for insurance or employment purposes, or pre-operatively. Ideally, every adult should have their blood pressure checked at intervals throughout life from the day they leave school. This would result in enormous reductions in both morbidity and mortality. Figure 4.4B (p.236) shows a possible protocol for screening.

Hypertension may be diagnosed as a result of a measurement of blood pressure taken when a patient goes to see a doctor complaining of headache. The myth has therefore grown up that hypertension causes headache. This is not so, although malignant hypertension, which is associated with raised intracranial pressure, usually does.

Hypertension often precipitates angina in patients with ischaemic heart disease. It is not unusual for it to be discovered when a patient presents with chest pain.

If hypertension is diagnosed early, as a result of a routine test, there will be no abnormal physical findings. A healthy heart can comfortably sustain moderately raised systemic pressure for a considerable period without developing significant hypertrophy of the left ventricle and target organs will also be unaffected.

If it is severe or long-standing, you may find LVH: on clinical examination and on ECG; retinal changes (see below) and evidence of renal damage (e.g. albumenuria; uraemia).

WHAT SHOULD YOU DO?

These questions need to be answered:
(1)   Is the blood pressure truly raised; if so, by how much?
(2)   Is it due to benign essential hypertension or is it secondary to an underlying cause?
(3)   Are there any complications?

Then the following procedures should be carried out for *all* patients.

Blood pressure

– Take blood pressure at least 3 times on different days. This should be done, no matter how high the initial reading, otherwise a baseline is never established.
– A standard routine should be adopted by every practice: this is usually to measure pressure in the right arm with the with the patient sitting. The cuff should be placed with the bag over the front of the arm so that the pressure is applied over the brachial artery when it is inflated. It is then easier to arrange it so that the tubes come out of the top.

– If the patient has a fat arm, consider using a thigh cuff.

History

(1)   Take a careful history, looking for evidence of alternative diagnoses or complications:
      Ureteric colic
      Pyelitis
      Haematuria
      Chest pain
      Breathlessness
      Dementia
      Smoking
      Alcohol consumption
      Drugs: oral contraceptives, systemic steroids, other medication.

(2)   Ask if a normal blood pressure has ever been recorded (e.g. at employment or insurance medical or during pregnancy).

(3)   This is a good opportunity to check for anything which may influence the choice of treatment:
Smoking
Alcohol
Stress/personality type
Asthma
Family history of hypertension or ischaemic heart disease
Symptoms of peripheral vascular disease (intermittent claudication; Raynaud's phenomenon).

Examination

(1)   General appearance – note:
- weight;
- plethora;
- Cushinoid appearance;
- evidence of hyperthyroidism, hypothyroidism, anxiety, smoking, alcohol;
- pointers to coexistent atheroma: arcus senilis, xantholasma, tendon xanthomata peripheral vascular disease.

(2)   Cardiovascular system:
- BP three times (see above);
- take peripheral pulses including carotids;
- femoral pulses: are they delayed?
- optic fundi: (dilate the pupils if necessary):
  - Grade I: arterial thickening ('silver wiring') only;
  - Grade II: arterial thickening ('silver wiring'), tortuosity and A – V nipping;
  - Grade III: haemorrhages and exudates;
  - Grade IV: papilloedema as well as Grade III changes.

(3)   Heart:
- check cardiac impulse for LV+;
- listen carefully for aortic diastolic murmur of aortic regurgitation, especially if systolic hypertension with wide pulse pressure.

Investigations

(1)   Urine for albumen, glucose, cells, casts and culture.

(2)   Blood for FBC, urea and electrolytes, blood sugar and serum cholesterol.

(3)   ECG is usually normal when first seen. Severe, long-standing hypertension always causes left ventricular hypertrophy (LVH) eventually. Some people develop LVH at an early stage and they have a worse prognosis and should be treated more vigorously;
LVH on ECG (Figure 4.4A) is shown by:
  – S in V1 + R in V6 = 40 mm (40 small squares); or more
  – S – T segment changes and T wave inversion in leads I, II and V3 – 6.

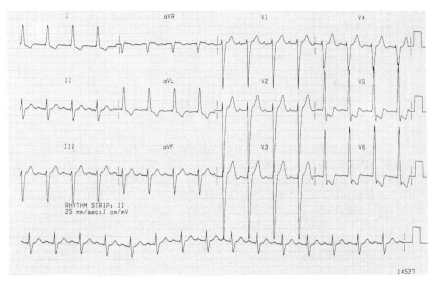

Figure 4.4A Left ventricular hypertrophy

(4)   Chest X-ray is usually normal. There may be dilatation of the aorta.

(5)   If there is a history of kidney disease, an IVP should also be done.

These investigations will:

(1)   Establish whether the patient has hypertension;

(2)   Discover whether it has had any effects on the fundi, kidneys or left ventricle;

(3)   Help to exclude other causes:
          Coarctation of the aorta (rib notching)
          Renal disease
          Conn's syndrome (low potassium)
          Cushing's syndrome (high sodium);

(4)   Identify complicating conditions such as diabetes, ischaemic heart disease, peripheral vascular disease, asthma, stress factors, smoking, alcohol.

HOW CAN HIGH BLOOD PRESSURE BE REDUCED?

More than in any other condition, the successful management of hypertension demands a partnership between the patient and the doctor. No advice will be followed nor drugs taken, if the patient fails to appreciate the point of it all. The doctor may think he is treating the patient but, in reality, the patient is (or is not) treating himself or herself with help from the doctor in the form of advice and/or prescription. There are several reasons why it is especially difficult for patients with hypertension to co-operate with their treatment:

(1)   There are no symptoms and so no immediate benefit can be expected.

(2)   Treatment often needs to start when the patient is quite young and the theoretical threat of some distant complication, such as stroke, seems very far off and unreal.

(3)   Side-effects, both real and imagined, are common, especially during the early stages of treatment.

(4)   Visits to the doctor for blood pressure checks and adjustments to drug dosage have to be frequent at first and may seem very irksome.

(5)   Young people, who feel fit, do not like to be constantly reminded that there is something wrong with them: taking medication reminds them every day.

(6)   Drug treatment has had a bad press and many people are understandably suspicious of it.

Once the diagnosis has been made, the initial interview with the patient is important. The future success of the treatment depends on it. The doctor needs to know as much from the patient as the patient from the doctor.

The details will depend on the individual and on whether the management is planned to include drugs.

The doctor needs to know

- What does the patient already know (or fear) about the condition and its treatment?
- Has he or she relatives or friends with hypertension?
- What does he feel about the idea of changing his lifestyle: stopping smoking, losing weight, taking exercise?
- Would he/could he cope with taking regular medication?
- Are there any special considerations necessary due to his work or leisure activities? Does he work as a pilot or HGV driver? Is he a mountaineer or parachutist in his spare time?

The patient needs to know

- What is hypertension?
- How bad is his hypertension?
- What will happen (a) without treatment and (b) with treatment?
- What is the treatment? How long will he have to take it?
- Will it have any side-effects? What are they?
- How often will he have to attend for check ups?
- Will it effect his work/prospects/leisure activities/sex life?

He may not think to ask all these questions but his need for information should be anticipated, as far as possible. This will save time and trouble in the long term by improving compliance.

He is not likely to take in the implications of all this at once, and it helps a great deal if he can be given time to consider his decision. After all, it is he who has to take the treatment: his responsibility. He is more likely to take it seriously if he feels it has been truly his own decision. A booklet or leaflet, repeating and enlarging on what the doctor has said, is useful but it cannot take the place of the initial explanation.

Non-drug treatment

This depends on the enthusiastic co-operation of the patient. It includes:

No smoking
Maintenance of correct weight
Regular exercise
Relaxation: formal/ daily   } FOR LIFE
Learning to deal with stress
Healthy diet.

These are good principles for everyone and they should certainly be recommended for anyone with:
- a family history of hypertension;
- occasional high blood pressure readings;
- a blood pressure towards the upper end of the normal range;
- confirmed hypertension.

A reduced salt intake is worth a trial for a few months as it may make a significant difference and render drug treatment unnecessary.

Even for those who need anti-hypertensive drugs, the general measures are important and can make a significant difference to the morbidity and mortality. Once drug treatment has been started, it is difficult for many people to continue with the non-drug measures. The temptation is to sit back and leave it to the drugs It is therefore helpful to get these general measures established before starting drugs.

Mild hypertension

Non-drug treatment should be given first for 2–3 months. This allows time for any temporary effects, such as transient worries, to pass, for the patient to get used to the general measures and for a steady base-line of readings to be recorded.

This may be all that is needed, particularly if the patient had a large number of changes to make and has indeed made them. If he is already a lean, active, relaxed, teetotal, non-smoker, then non-drug treatment will make little difference.

The decision as to whether drugs should be used for mild hypertension is not clear cut.

Women with mild hypertension benefit very little from drug treatment. If drugs are prescribed, it is better to use beta-blockers than thiazide diuretics.

Non-smoking men do benefit but the advantages can be easily outweighed by side-effects, by lack of enthusiasm, or poor compliance.

In smokers, the incidence of stroke is reduced by thiazides, although not by beta-blockers.

As a rough guide, drug treatment should be considered in:
- anyone with a diastolic pressure consistently over 100 mmHg;
- men;
- those with other risk factors (e.g. hyperlipidaemia, a bad family history);
- those who have already sustained damage to organs:
    - left ventricle: hypertrophy; failure;
    - brain: CVA; encephalopathy;
    - kidneys: renal impairment/failure.

Current research may make this whole area clearer.

Whether or not it is decided to use drug treatment for mild hypertension, long-term follow up is extremely important as the condition can progress and become more severe, with a corresponding increase in risk. The indications for and choice of treatment may then be different. See Chapter 5.3 p.324 for suggestions as to how long-term follow-up may be done.

Moderate and severe hypertension

Non-drug treatment, as for mild hypertension, is combined with drug treatment. This improves the efficacy of the drugs and allows dosage to be kept to a minimum.

The drugs commonly used are:
Thiazide diuretics
Beta-blockers
Calcium-channel blockers
Angiotensin converting enzyme inhibitors
Methyldopa
Peripheral vasodilators: hydralazine; alpha-blockers.

It is useful to have a standard regime which is used unless there are particular reasons not to in an individual case.

This is an area which lends itself particularly well to the drawing up of a practice protocol. Here is a suggested plan for an uncomplicated patient with normal renal function. First, here are the general principles:
- Allow 4 weeks between each stage.
- Check for side-effects at each stage.
- Stop increments when BP is controlled.
- Aim for a diastolic pressure between 90 and 100 mmHg.
- Try to avoid taking the blood pressure as soon as the patient sits down: a more reliable reading is obtained by waiting a few minutes.

The plan will include the following stages:

Pre-treatment: three readings at intervals; examination and investigations as above (p.228).

Stage 1: Beta-blocker (e.g. atenolol 50 mg daily).

Stage 2: add thiazide diuretic (e.g. bendrofluazide 2.5 mg daily).

Stage 3: add calcium-channel blocker (e.g. nifedipine retard 20 mg twice a day).

Note: there is no point in increasing the dose of beta-blocker or giving more diuretic than this. In fact, smaller doses of diuretic may be equally effective.

Stage 4: check blood urea and electrolytes; add vasodilator (e.g. hydralazine 25 mg twice daily) or alpha-blocker such as prazosin, starting with 1 mg at night and increasing gradually to maximum of 2 g daily in divided doses; take blood pressure standing as well as sitting from now on.

Stage 5: if patient male, increase dose of hydralazine to 25 mg three times a day. If female, go to next stage.

Stage 6: consider referral or replace hydralazine by ACE inhibitor (e.g. captopril 12.5 mg twice daily, increasing to 25 mg twice daily if necessary). Check blood urea before first dose and after 2 – 4 weeks.

This plan should be varied in the following circumstances:
- in smokers, it is better to start with a thiazide – i.e. reverse order of stages 1 and 2
- if beta-blockers are contra-indicated (history of asthma, peripheral vascular disease or heart failure), start with a diuretic and then add a calcium-channel blocker.

The patient should be seen monthly for the first 2–3 months. Once the blood pressure is controlled, the patient need not be seen so often but a long-term plan should be agreed. Follow up can be shared between the doctor and the practice nurse, following agreed, written guidelines (see below).

If control is good, visits can reasonably be as much as 6 months apart, perhaps alternating between nurse and doctor.

After a few years of good control, it may be possible to reduce the dose of drugs gradually and even to stop them altogether. Monitoring of the blood pressure should be continued indefinitely.

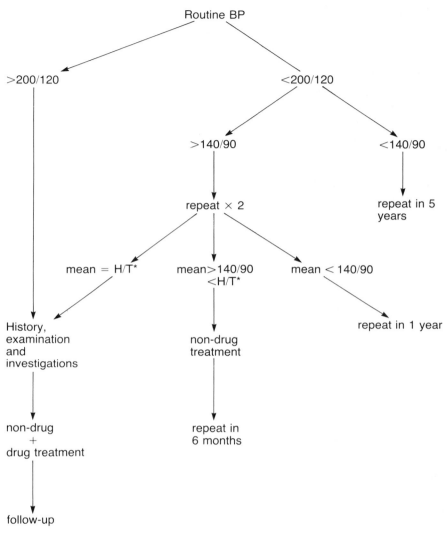

Figure 4.4B Protocol for hypertension screening
* depends on age: see p.221

Guidelines for long-term follow-up of hypertensive patients by nurses.

1. Weight, lifestyle, smoking

2. Side effects of medication

3. BP sitting (standing also if over 60 or on vasodilator); repeat after a few days if in doubt.

4. Refer to doctor if pressure outside agreed range (to be stated for each patient)

4.5
Arrhythmias

WHAT ARE THEY?

Arrhythmias arise when there are departures from the normal pattern of electrical conduction and myocardial contraction. They cause abnormalities of heart rate or of co-ordination of myocardial contraction or both. (For a description of the normal pattern of conduction and contraction, see Chapter 1.4 p.31)

In *abnormalities of rate*, the heart beats too fast, too slowly or alternates between the two. Examples are atrial fibrillation, heart block and the brady-tachy syndrome.

In *abnormalities of co-ordination*, the different parts of the myocardium fail to contract in an orderly and normal sequence. For instance, in atrial fibrillation, the atria do not contract effectively at all; in heart block, the atria contract but not necessarily during ventricular diastole and so the normal pattern is disturbed.

In the last two examples, the rate is usually also disturbed.

Arrhythmias result from abnormal pacemakers, abnormal conduction or from a combination of the two.

Abnormal (ectopic) pacemakers

(1)   The depolarisation wave arises from an alternative pacemaker in:
   – the atrium (supraventricular ectopic beats)
   – the junctional tissue (A – V node)
   – the ventricle (ventricular ectopic beats).

If this happens because the sinus node fails or the depolarisation wave is not conducted, the resulting rhythm is slower, e.g. the idioventricular rate of complete heart block.

This may be a stable situation, in which there is a single ectopic focus or multiple pacemakers in different sites may alternate (multifocal beats).

The S–A node may continue to function so that some normally conducted beats are produced.

If the sinus node rate is slow, the natural rate of other tissue may result in extra beats (escape beats); an ectopic pacemaker can only take over from the sinus node if its rate is faster. If the sinus rate is normal, arrhythmias may result from increased excitability of the myocardium such as may be caused by sympathetic activity, electrolyte imbalance, ventricular dilatation, ischaemia, drugs.

Abnormal conduction

(1)   Reduced rate of conduction:
       – A–V block
       – bundle branch block.

(2)   Additional aberrant conduction through abnormal pathways:
       – Wolff–Parkinson–White syndrome.

The combination of abnormal pacemakers and abnormal conduction

These can give rise to a large number of possible combinations and varieties of defect. We will not attempt to describe all these complex patterns but will consider only the main groups:

(1)   *Variations of sinus rhythm*: the sequence and pattern of electrical activity is normal but the rate is not:

       – sinus arrhythmia (Figure 4.5A): this is not an abnormal condition. The heart rate increases with inspiration and decreases with expiration due to variations in vagal tone with respiration;

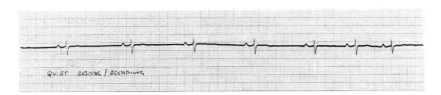

Figure 4.5A ECG: sinus arrhythmia

       – sinus tachycardia: this is normal in every way except that the rate is more than 100/min; has many causes including: anxiety, fever, haemorrhage, hyperthyroidism;

       – sinus bradycardia: this is normal in every way except that the rate is less than 60/min; is normal in certain individuals, especially

239

athletes; has many causes, including hypothyroidism, hypothermia, raised intra-cranial pressure, beta-blockers and acute myocardial infarction; may need pacing, if output seriously reduced.

(2)   *Abnormal atrial rhythms*:
   – paroxysmal supraventricular tachycardia: this arises from an ectopic atrial pacemaker; if the pacemaker is near the A – V node, the P wave is hidden in the subsequent QRS complex and will not be identifiable; no known cause but trigger factors (e.g.coffee) may be identified;

   – junctional, or nodal, rhythm is the name given to one which arises from an ectopic pacemaker near the A – V node. The rate is normal but no P waves are seen on the ECG;

   – atrial flutter: this is a rapid atrial rate, 300/minute, with a variable degree of A – V block; the block may be constant, producing a regular rate, or varying, producing an irregular pulse; usually associated with underlying heart disease;

   – In atrial fibrillation, atrial contraction is lost and replaced by a continuous trembling motion, which has no effect on emptying the atria; the A – V node can conduct only a proportion of the huge number of impulses which bombard it from the atria; the ventricles beat as a result of those depolarisation waves, which are conducted through the A – V node; the QRS complexes are normal in shape, because they result from normal A – V conduction but they are irregular; caused by mitral stenosis, ischaemic heart disease, hyperthyroidism, hypertension, cardiomyopathy and 'lone' (idiopathic) fibrillation.

(3)   *Ventricular rhythms*:

   – arise from two main sets of circumstances:

(a)   Depolarisation waves fail to reach the ventricles via the A – V node, either because of A – V block or because the sinus node has stopped producing impulses and no alternative (ectopic) atrial pacemaker has taken over its role. This is third degree (complete) heart block.
       In this situation, the ventricles beat at their own (idio ventricular) rate, which is very slow.
       This can be an established situation or can occur in bouts varying from a few beats to a prolonged attack.

(b)   A ventricular focus produces an electrical impulse, causing depolarisation, before the one conducted from the sinus node.

    This can occur as a single event, producing a ventricular extrasystole, or as a prolonged run of ventricular ectopic beats, which is then called ventricular tachycardia.

    The terms, ectopic beat and extrasystole, have the same meaning.

(4)   *Heart block (atrioventricular block)*: this is caused by delay or complete interruption of conduction of impulses from the atria to the ventricles through the A – V node.

  – In first degree heart block (Figure 4.5B): the delay has the effect of prolonging the conduction time through the A – V node, causing an increase in the P – R interval beyond 0.2 sec (five small squares).

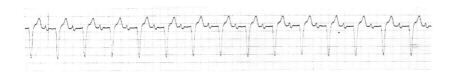

Figure 4.5B First degree heart block

  – second degree heart block is subdivided into two types:

    type 1 (Wenckebach; Figure 4.5C): the conduction delay increases in successive beats until one impulse fails to be conducted and a beat is dropped. The number of beats in each cycle varies.

    type 2 (Figure 4.5D): some depolaristion waves are conducted and some are not.

    There may be a regular relationship in which, for instance, every second or every third impulse is blocked: 2:1 or 3:1 block or the relationship may vary.

    All the ventricular contractions result from normally conducted depolarisation waves so that there is a P wave before each QRS complex, although a QRS complex does not follow every P wave.

  – third degree heart block is described above under ventricular rhythms.

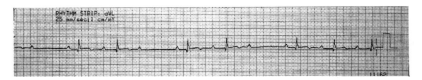

Figure 4.5C Wenckebach: the T-wave inversion is due to an inferior infarct

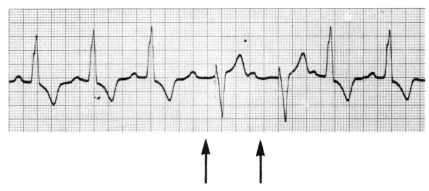

Figure 4.5D Type 2 second degree heart block. This patient is fitted with a demand ventricular pacemaker (VVD). The arrows point to paced beats triggered by the failure of the depolarisation wave to be conducted

WHAT CAUSES ARRHYTHMIAS?

(1) Congenital abnormalities in the specialised conducting tissue:
       e.g. heart block;
              Wolff – Parkinson – White syndrome.

(2) Diseases:
       e.g. IHD (most arrhythmias)
              Mitral stenosis (atrial fibrillation)
              Hyperthyroidism (atrial fibrillation)
              Carcinoma of lung (atrial fibrillation)
              Infections: diphtheria, rheumatic fever, myocarditis.

(3) Toxins: e.g. alcohol, smoking, caffeine (tea, coffee), drugs, especially digoxin.

(4) Electrolyte imbalance: e.g. potassium depletion or excess.

In many patients, no cause is found.

WHAT HAPPENS?

Symptoms and problems arise from arrhythmias:
(1)   if the rate is very fast
(2)   if the rate is very slow
(3)   if A – V contraction is incordinate
(4)   in atrial fibrillation
The symptoms will depend on the type of arrhythmia and on the health of the
myocardium (Table 4.5A):

Table 4.5A Symptoms of arrhythmias

	Healthy myocardium	Unhealthy myocardium
FAST	Palpitations Dizzy spells	Palpitations Angina Heart failure
SLOW	Stokes – Adams attacks	Stokes – Adams attacks Heart failure
AF	Palpitations Dizzy spells	Palpitations Heart failure Emboli Angina

(1)   *If rate is very fast:*
– Filling time is reduced, causing reduced cardiac output: makes the patient
   feel faint; may cause heart failure.
– The oxygen requirements of the myocardium are increased: if the
   coronary arteries are narrowed, this may cause angina.
– Ventricular fibrillation may follow, especially if the rate is excessive, the
   attack prolonged, the myocardium irritable or, above all, if the
   tachycardia is ventricular.

(2)   *If rate is very slow:*
– The patient may lose consciousness (Stokes – Adams attack).
– Cardiac output is reduced and may cause heart failure.

(3)   *If A – V contraction is incoordinate:*
– The contribution of atrial contraction to ventricular filling is lost, reducing
   cardiac efficiency and increasing the amount of work required for a given
   output.

- Cannon waves may be seen in the neck veins when the right atrium contracts against the closed tricuspid valve.

(4)   *In atrial fibrillation:*
- Turbulence and inadequate emptying allow clots to form in the atria. These can form emboli. On the left side, this can have disastrous results.

Hidden danger

Type 2 second degree heart block may be associated with periods of complete heart block. There are likely to be no symptoms of the initial arrhythmia. The first sign of complete heart block may be fatal.

WHICH IS IT?

Paroxysmal supra-ventricular tachycardia

In supraventricular tachycardia (SVT) (see Figure 4.5E):

- The patient likely to be young and fit;

- The arrhythmia occurs in attacks and the attacks start suddenly; may stop suddenly or gradually;
- The rate is 140–220 and regular;

- The patient is well between attacks and not much incapacitated by them.

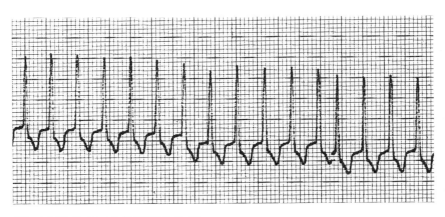

Figure 4.5E Supraventricular tachycardia

- ECG is normal between attacks:
  during attack the rate is 140–220; regular;
  P waves, if present, precede QRS;
  QRS in aVR always negative;
  QRS axis normal.
  (If rate is very fast and aberrant conduction, it may be difficult to distinguish from ventricular tachycardia.)

Atrial fibrillation

Atrial fibrillation (AF) (Figure 4.5F) is less common than SVT.

- The patient is usually older.

- It may occur in attacks; the patient may feel awful during attack; the attack starts suddenly.

- The rate is 100–150 and irregular.

- The attack is more likely to be prolonged (providing opportunity to obtain ECG during attack).

- The AF eventually becomes the established rhythm, either from the start or after many attacks.

- The ECG may be normal between attacks.
  During attack, or when AF established:
  No P waves (they may or may not be replaced by a jagged pattern between QRS complexes)
  QRS complexes normal in shape but irregular.

(AF with a slow atrial rate may cause a lumpy wave, which may look like atrial flutter, but the QRS complexes are always irregular in atrial fibrillation.)

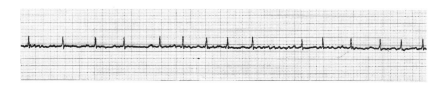

Figure 4.5F Atrial fibrillation

Atrial flutter

Atrial flutter (Figure 4.5G) is usually associated with underlying heart disease.

– It may occur in attacks.

– It does not cause symptoms unless very fast or cardiac reserve limited.

– The ECG has regular P waves usually called flutter waves (saw-toothed pattern) at 300/minute;
each QRS is preceded by P wave;
QRS complexes regular, if block stays the same;
if block varying, QRS complexes separated by varying number of flutter waves.

(a)

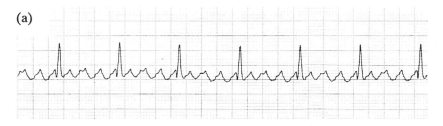

(b) V1

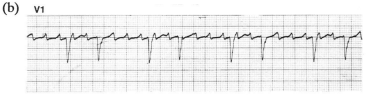

Figure 4.5G Atrial flutter (a) regular 4:1 block, ventricular rate 75/min (clinically indistinguishable from sinus rhythm)
(b) varying block with irregular ventricular rate

Ventricular tachycardia

This is a run of more than three ventricular ectopic beats (Figure 4.5H) (the number is arbitrary and experts differ).

– It is rare in young, healthy subjects.

– It is usually associated with heart disease so that attacks cause angina, dizzyness and heart failure very soon.

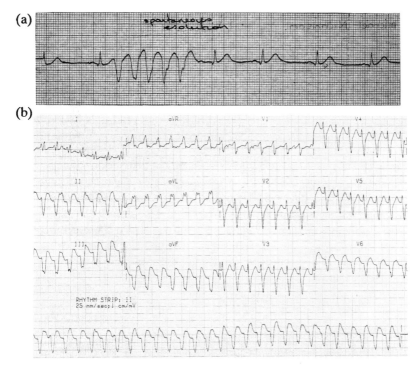

Figure 4.5H Ventricular tachycardia (a) a short run of VT with spontaneous resolution (b) established VT

- Attacks may be short (diagnosable only by ambulatory monitoring) or prolonged.

- The rate is 110–220 and regular.

- The ECG:
  between attacks: usually shows signs of underlying disease
  during attack: no P waves or independent P waves at a slower rate than the QRS complexes;
  QRS complexes broad and bizarre;
  QRS in aVR positive;
  QRS axis may be grossly abnormal.

Table 4.5B should assist differentiation of VT from SVT when there are no P waves.

Table 4.5B Comparing supraventricular (SVT) with ventricular tachycardia (VT)

SVT	VT
QRS in aVR negative	QRS in aVR positive
Normal axis	Bizarrely abnormal axis
Narrow QRS complexes	Broad QRS complexes
(unless aberrant conduction)	
Always regular	Usually regular
May be stopped by vagal stimulation	Unaffected by vagal stimulation

Ventricular extrasystoles

These are isolated ventricular (Figure 4.5I) ectopic beats. The beat following the extrasystole is delayed (compensatory pause) and the following, conducted, beat is of greater volume and therefore more forceful. This is what the patient notices.

It is often described clearly as a missed beat followed by a strong one. They occur in healthy people and are then of no significance.

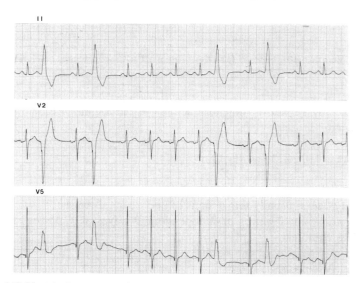

Figure 4.5I Ventricular extrasystoles

Heart block

First degree heart block: This causes no symptoms nor abnormal physical signs. The ECG has P–R interval greater than 0.2 sec (five small squares); rate normal.

Second degree heart block: This often causes no symptoms but patient may notice missed beats. Patients with type 2 may give a history of syncope, suggesting episodes of third degree block. (For ECG see p.35.)

Third degree heart block: This is commonest in elderly people with conducting system disease but may affect apparently healthy people who have a congenital abnormality of the conducting system. It may occur intermittently so that the patient appears normal when seen. It causes attacks of dizzyness or cardiac syncope (Stokes–Adams attacks). The patient feels himself losing consciousness (unlike the sudden drop attacks typical of senile epilepsy, which occur without warning).

The ECG shows regular P waves at physiological rate; regular QRS complexes of normal shape, slower than P waves; no relationship whatsoever between P waves and QRS complexes.

Note: that this is probably the second most missed cardiac diagnosis (the first is left ventricular failure). It should be borne in mind in anyone who suffers from dizzy turns or fainting attacks.

WHAT DO YOU DO?

The aims of management

(1)   Accurate diagnosis of the arrhythmia.

(2)   Identification and treatment of complicating conditions, such as electrolyte imbalance, heart failure or angina.

(3)   Identification of any underlying cause, such as hyperthyroidism, mitral stenosis or drug toxicity.

(4)   Control of symptoms.

(5)   Prevention of complications.

Every patient suspected of having a significant arrhythmia should have:
  – A physical examination

- An ECG
- Other tests or referral, if needed, to achieve the above aims.

If an arrhythmia occurs as a complication of acute myocardial infarction, the patient should be admitted to hospital.

Paroxysmal SVT

An ECG taken during an attack is useful confirmation of the diagnosis but is seldom possible. Ambulatory monitoring can be used but the condition is so benign that it is not usually justified.

An ECG taken between attacks is useful to identify other abnormalities, e.g. Wolff–Parkinson–White syndrome. Unless the symptoms are really trivial, thyroid function tests should be done.

Healthy people usually need nothing more than reassurance.

If attacks are a nuisance:
- try vagal stimulation:
  - Valsalva (must be demonstrated);
  - drop down quickly onto one knee as if to do up shoe;
- avoid possible triggers: tea, coffee, alcohol, stress.

If attacks are really obtrusive, drugs may have to be considered:
- digoxin first, as long as the diagnosis is beyond reasonable doubt (dangerous in VT);
- beta-blocker can be used with digoxin or on its own;
- verapamil can be useful but must not be given with a beta-blocker or digoxin;
- disopyramide, quinidine or amiodarone may be tried in refractory cases (consider referral).

Atrial fibrillation

Hyperthyroidism is such a common, easily missed and treatable condition that it is worth doing thyroid function tests on every patient with atrial fibrillation. If the cause is obscure, a chest X-ray should be taken to exclude bronchial carcinoma.

The main risk of atrial fibrillation is systemic emboli. Therefore, anticoagulant treatment should be considered in all patients unless:
- there is a clinical contra-indication, such as a bleeding diathesis; active peptic ulcer;
- the left atrium is small and mitral valve healthy.

If the ventricular rate is uncomfortably fast, the patient should be digitalised, the dose being adjusted to achieve a ventricular rate of 60 – 80/min.

Atrial flutter

- Cardioversion to sinus rhythm with DC shock should always be considered.
- Digoxin slows the rate but may encourage the rhythm to convert to atrial fibrillation. Sometimes, it may revert to sinus rhythm if treatment is stopped.

Ventricular tachycardia

The patient is likely to be in or attending hospital. If persistent, VT is an emergency as it may change to ventricular fibrillation at any time. It therefore needs immediate treatment by DC shock. If intermittent, an antiarrhythmic drug, such as amiodarone, should be given.

Extrasystoles need no treatment

Heart block

First degree heart block: No treatment is required unless the cause needs treatment, e.g. digoxin toxicity.

Second degree heart block: Type 1: no treatment is required unless the cause needs treatment, e.g. myocardial infarction.

Type 2: because of the hidden danger of complete heart block previously referred to (p.244), these patients should be referred for consideration of pacing.

Third degree heart block: These patients nearly always need a pacemaker.

WHO TO REFER?

Patients:
- with any arrhythmia following acute myocardial infarction;
- in whom the diagnosis is difficult;
- with type 2 second degree heart block;

- with third degree heart block;
- with any arrhythmia causing symptoms, which are difficult to control;
- with atrial fibrillation for consideration of anticoagulation;
- with ventricular tachycardia.

PACEMAKERS

What are they?

A pacemaker is an electronic device which delivers a stimulating impulse to the myocardium in a prearranged way. A permanent pacemaker is made of inert material and is inserted in the subcutaneous tissue just below the clavicle, usually the left. There are several different types and they can be programmed in different ways depending on the needs of the patient and the limitations of cost.

A wire (sometimes two) leads from the box into the right heart via a vein. There is an electrode, sometimes several, on the end of the wire, which is embedded in the myocardium. Some are unipolar, the second pole being on the box itself. Others are bipolar, with both poles at the tip of the wire.

Figure 4.5J shows a chest X-ray with pacemaker *in situ*.

How do they work?

All pacemakers are described by three letters (Table 4.5C).

The first stands for the chamber paced.
The next stands for the chamber sensed.
The third for the mode of response.

Table 4.5C Coding of pacemakers

Chamber paced	Chamber sensed	Mode of response
A = atrium	O = none	O = not applicable
V = ventricle	A = atrium	I = inhibited
D = both	V = ventricle	T = triggered
	D = both	D = both inhibited
		and triggered

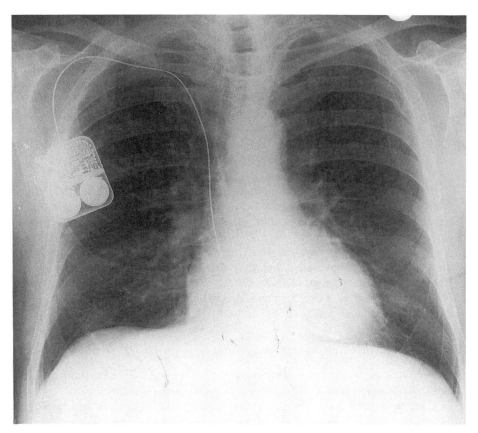

Figure 4.5J Chest X-ray with pacemaker *in situ*

In the simplest type of pacemaker, a single wire ends in a single electrode which is embedded in the right ventricle. It is set to produce an impulse at a fixed rate. It is known as an VOO pacemaker: the chamber paced is the ventricle (V), no chamber is being sensed (O) and therefore the last letter does not apply (O).

This is not an ideal system. The problems are that:

(1)   The pacemaker is unaffected by spontaneous activity of the heart so that there is a risk that an impulse will arrive just as the refractory period of the previous spontaneous beat is ending. This may precipitate ventricular tachycardia – the 'R-on-T' effect.

(2)   Atrial contraction is not co-ordinated with ventricular contraction so that, when the atria contract, the A–V valves may be closed. If there

is retrograde conduction from the ventricles to the atria via the A – V node, with every paced beat, then the atria will contract against closed A – V valves in every beat.

This causes blood to flow backwards from the atria into the main veins. When the A – V valves do open, it takes a little time for the flow to reverse and ventricular filling is slow to start. This, added to the loss of the contribution of atrial contraction to ventricular filling, means that the ventricular end diastolic volume is reduced and cardiac output seriously compromised. This gives rise to the 'pacemaker syndrome' in which the patient feels dizzy and confused due to a low cardiac output.

In a VVI pacemaker, spontaneous activity of the ventricle, resulting either from a normally conducted sinus beat or from an ectopic beat, inhibits the pacemaker so that there is no risk of an R-on-T beat. Asynchronous atrial activity remains a problem.

More complex pacemakers, which overcome both the problems described above, have been developed but they are expensive and not widely used. Pacemakers in current general use do not allow for an increase in heart rate on exercise. Work is in progress to address this problem.

When are they used?

Pacemakers are used on a temporary basis for transient arrhythmias after myocardial infarction.

The main indication for *permanent* pacing is symptomatic bradycardia, usually due to heart block or sick sinus syndrome. The symptoms are:

Lightheadedness, dizzyness	Poor exercise tolerance
Confusion	Angina
Syncope fatigue, exhaustion	Heart failure.

Other indications are:
- heart rate less than 40/min, even if asymptomatic;
- sinus bradycardia with frequent ventricular ectopic (escape) beats;
- episodes of asystole of 3 sec or more on ambulatory monitoring (Figure 4.5K);
- type 2 second degree heart block with two or more consecutive P waves blocked (Figure 4.5L).

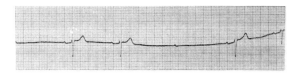

Figure 4.5K Bradycardia due to slow sinus rate and intermittent A – V block

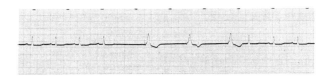

Figure 4.5L Sinus arrest: ventricular pacing showing pacing spikes

4.6
Valvular Disease

In the past, rheumatic carditis was responsible for the vast majority of valvular disease. Acute rheumatism continued to be common, in the UK, until the mid-1950s. There is still a large pool of patients, over 40, who suffered rheumatic fever as children and who now have chronic rheumatic heart disease.

Acute rheumatism is now rare in developed countries but common in developing countries and in immigrants. It is important to diagnose promptly and the possibility should be kept in mind in any child or adolescent with flitting arthralgia and malaise.

WHAT IS VALVE DISEASE?

Congenital, inflammatory or degenerative change in a valve, which causes it to fail to open or close fully. Chronic infection of an abnormal valve (subacute bacterial endocarditis; SBE) destroys the valve and leads to the formation of vegetations, which break off as emboli.

WHAT HAPPENS?

The effects are:
(1)   Haemodynamic
(2)   Electrical
(3)   Embolic.

(1)   Haemodynamic

Obstruction to the outflow of a ventricle causes pressure overload, which results in hypertrophy (Figure 4.6A) of the muscle but no dilatation. The walls of the ventricle are thicker than normal but the volume is unchanged.

Regurgitant ventricular outflow valves cause volume overload, which leads to hypertrophy and dilatation of the ventricle (Figure 4.6A). The volume of the ventricle is greater than usual but the walls are of normal thickness.

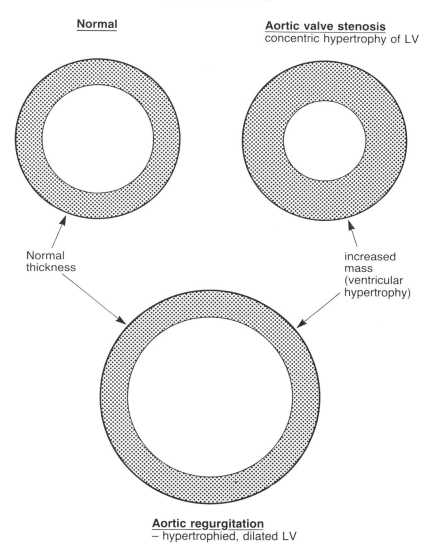

Figure 4.6A Ventricular hypertrophy in obstructive and high-output disease

The total mass of ventricular muscle is the same in both these situations.
As long as there is no heart failure:
– obstruction by a stenotic A – V valve leads to atrial dilatation and hypertrophy on that side;
– obstruction by a stenotic ventricular outflow tract valve leads to ventricular hypertrophy, with wall thickening but no dilatation;

– back flow in a regurgitant A – V valve causes atrial dilatation and ventricular hypertrophy and dilatation;

– back flow in a regurgitant outflow tract valve leads to ventricular hypertrophy and dilatation but little or no wall thickening.

(2)   *Electrical*

An example of this is atrial fibrillation in mitral valve disease. The left atrium is dilated, the flow turbulent and emptying incomplete so that thrombi form, especially within the atrial appendage.

(3)   *Embolic*

There are two examples of embolic effects:
emboli from thrombus in a dilated, turbulant atrium: systemic on left; pulmonary on right;
septic emboli from vegetations on a valve in SBE: into the systemic circulation (from the left side of the heart) or to the lungs (from the right).

HOW DO YOU FIND OUT ABOUT VALVE DISEASE?

Diseased valves come to light because of murmurs or symptoms.

Murmurs

A murmur may be found during medical examination:
–   Routine well-baby check
–   School, employment, insurance medical
–   Ante-natal booking.

Systolic murmurs are of two basic types:
(1)   Those due to obstruction of a stenosed outflow tract valve or excessive flow through a normal outflow tract. These are called ejection murmurs and are diamond-shaped when drawn (Figure 4.6B).
       They occur in aortic and pulmonary stenosis and in large shunts, when there is increased flow through these valves.

258

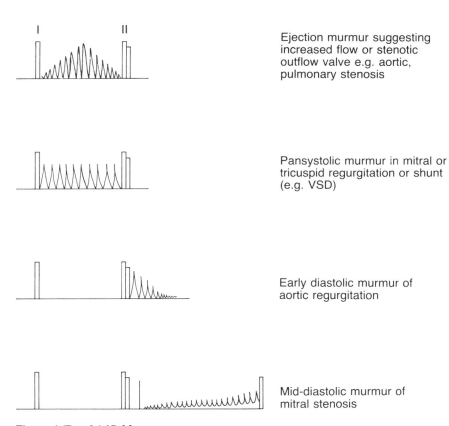

Ejection murmur suggesting increased flow or stenotic outflow valve e.g. aortic, pulmonary stenosis

Pansystolic murmur in mitral or tricuspid regurgitation or shunt (e.g. VSD)

Early diastolic murmur of aortic regurgitation

Mid-diastolic murmur of mitral stenosis

Figures 4.6B and 4.6C Murmurs

(2)   those due to backflow through a regurgitant A – V valve or flow through a septal defect (Figure 4.6C).

Diastolic murmurs are always pathological. The most important are heard in aortic regurgitation and mitral stenosis.

Symptoms caused by diseased valves

(1)   Aortic stenosis:
                angina
                syncope
                sudden death.

(2)   Aortic regurgitation:
          left heart failure.

(3)   Mitral stenosis/regurgitation:
          palpitations (AF)
          arterial embolism
          heart failure.

We will discuss only aortic and mitral valve disease because tricuspid and pulmonary valve disease are relatively uncommon.

4.6.1   AORTIC STENOSIS

What is it?

Narrowing of the left ventricular outflow tract: the normal valve area is $3-4$ cm^2. Resistance to flow occurs when the area is reduced to between 1.5 and 1.0 cm^2 and there is a gradient between the aorta and the ventricle during systole.
     It can be caused by:
     – disease of the aortic valve (aortic valve stenosis)
     OR
     – thickening of the muscle just below the valve (sub-valvar stenosis).
These are clinically very similar.

What causes it?

Aortic valve stenosis can be due to:
(1)   congenital heart disease, i.e. narrowed from birth;
(2)   rheumatic heart disease, with fusion of diseased cusps;
(3)   secondary, degenerative disease in a congenital bicuspid valve;
(4)   secondary, degenerative disease in a normal, tricuspid valve.
Aortic sub-valvar stenosis is described on p.265.

What happens?

All stenotic aortic valves calcify in time but the term 'calcific aortic stenosis' is sometimes used to describe those in which the calcification is part of the primary process (i.e. (3) and (4) in the causes listed above). The valve is calcified in anyone over 40 with stenosis. 95% of rheumatic aortic stenosis occurs together with mitral stenosis.

In congenital and rheumatic heart disease, the narrowing is associated with fusion of the cusps. The area of the outflow tract is therefore fixed and does not alter with changes in pressure or flow.

In the two secondary degenerative diseases, (3) and (4), the narrowing is caused by rigidity of the valve cusps. The cusps are free right up to the aortic ring and the outflow tract area can be increased if the pressure through it increases. The stenosis is, therefore, variable.

The main symptoms are:

Angina	Breathlessness
Syncope	Sudden death.

They seldom occur until the valve opening is less than 1 cm^2 in area and sometimes not until it is much more severe than this.

During exercise, the peripheral resistance is reduced, but, because of the narrowed left ventricular outflow tract, the cardiac output cannot be increased enough to maintain the blood pressure. This is why, in people with aortic stenosis, syncope and sudden death typically occur on exertion. Competitive and strenuous sport should be avoided.

CAMEO

Stephen Purchase is 38 and a university lecturer. He had no symptoms until he was playing in a cricket match and collapsed when running. He recovered quickly but a medical check revealed aortic valve stenosis. His diseased valve was replaced by a mechanical one and he is now fit and well, although he will have to take warfarin for the rest of his life.

CAMEO

Annie Melville is 87 and has been extremely fit until the last six months during which she has experienced increasing breathlessness on exertion. She is now confined to her flat and can barely move from one room to another. She has had two attacks of breathlessness, which have woken her at night and which were very frightening. She has recently found that she needs to sleep propped up on 3 or 4 pillows. She has been found to have severe aortic stenosis and is on the waiting list for valvuloplasty.

Of every 1000 babies, four are born with bicuspid aortic valves:
- one third function normally throughout life;
- one third develop predominant aortic stenosis;
- one third develop predominant aortic regurgitation.

In most people with bicuspid valves who develop disease, there is a mixture of stenosis and regurgitation.

The disease develops in the 6th, 7th and 8th decades. Degeneration of normal (tricuspid) valves occurs in the 8th and 9th decades.

Aortic stenosis causes massive left ventricular hypertrophy. The volume of the ventricle remains normal but the thickness of the walls increases.

The left ventricular muscle can become ischaemic without coronary artery disease. This is because:

(1)   systole is prolonged and diastole correspondingly short so that the time available for coronary perfusion is reduced.

(2)   the requirements of the hugely increased muscle mass are greater than normal.

Calcified (sclerotic) valves can cause very loud murmurs without significant stenosis.

Not all diseased aortic valves, even those with some degree of narrowing, progress to cause significant stenosis, requiring surgical intervention.

How do you know?

Anyone found to have a loud ejection murmur at the apex and the base of the heart AND anyone who develops angina or left heart failure should have a full examination, ECG and chest X-ray.

If significant aortic stenosis is present, these will reveal:

- Low cardiac output with poor peripheral perfusion, small pulse (typically slow-rising) and low pulse pressure.

- Left ventricular hypertrophy: on palpation of cardiac impulse; on ECG.

- A soft second heart sound.

- An ejection click, just after the second sound in the aortic area.

- Ejection, systolic murmur at the apex, in the aortic area, radiating into the neck. A systolic thrill may be felt in the aortic area and over the carotid arteries.

– Post-stenotic dilatation of the ascending aorta on chest X-ray.
   Calcification in the valve may be seen on a lateral view.
   There is no left ventricular dilatation in pure aortic stenosis so the left
   ventricle may not appear enlarged on the chest X-ray.

Figure 4.6D shows the aortic ejection murmur with ejection click and soft
second sound.

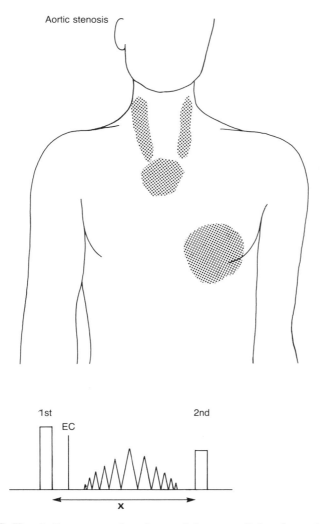

Figure 4.6D The ejection murmur of aortic stenosis is most easily heard over the sternum and
2nd right intercostal space with the patient leaning forward. It is also heard at the apex and
radiates into the neck. It is sometimes accompanied by a thrill

What do you do?

Sudden death may be the first indication of the presence of aortic stenosis and so it is important to refer patients for a cardiological opinion without waiting for symptoms to develop. The risk of sudden death is greatly increased if the patient is experiencing breathlessness, indicating left ventricular failure.

Early diagnosis is not as difficult as it sounds, as most people have their chests examined from time to time and the murmur of aortic stenosis is usually loud and obvious, as long as the doctor always keeps it in mind. It can be heard well with the patient sitting or standing; best leaning forward in a chair.

The initial referral for assessment is best made when the diagnosis is first suspected. The cardiologist will probably monitor the progress of the disease at very long intervals, perhaps seeing the patient every 3 years or so, if the condition appears stable.

Most patients with symptoms from aortic stenosis will be advised to have an operation. The timing of surgical intervention in asymptomatic patients is a matter for fine judgement, balancing the risk of sudden death against the risks of operation.

Drug treatment of angina associated with aortic stenosis presents real difficulties. Reduction of afterload, for example by a calcium-channel blocker, does not help and may reduce peripheral perfusion with disastrous results. Any drug which depresses myocardial contractility is likely to precipitate LV failure.

Surgical treatment

(1)   Valvotomy: mainly in children.

(2)   Valve replacement:
  – with mechanical valve: long-lasting but need life-long anti-coagulants;
  – with homograft (from pig): needs replacing after 5–10 years but no need for long-term anticoagulants and therefore suitable in elderly patients.

(3)   Balloon valvuloplasty: recently introduced with some success.

If successful surgical treatment is undertaken before the patient develops heart failure, left ventricular function can return to normal.

The most important part of long-term care is the prevention of SBE, although it is rare. All patients with aortic valve disease should be advised of the risks and take the precautions spelled out in Chapter 4.8. They should not be given antibiotics without clear indication and consideration of the possibility of SBE.

4.6.2 AORTIC SUB-VALVAR STENOSIS

What causes it?

It is part of hypertrophic obstructive cardiomyopathy (HOCM), in which the muscle of the left ventricular outflow tract thickens and narrows the passage, especially during systole, when the muscle contracts (Figure 4.6E).

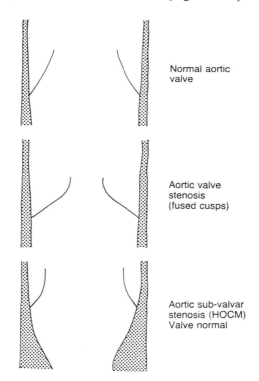

Normal aortic valve

Aortic valve stenosis (fused cusps)

Aortic sub-valvar stenosis (HOCM) Valve normal

Figure 4.6E Aortic stenosis

What happens?

The symptoms and signs are similar to aortic valve stenosis. It is a relentlessly progressive disease but advances at widely differing rates and it is reasonable to give patients a hopeful, if guarded, prognosis. There is the same risk of sudden death as in aortic valve stenosis. Competitive and strenuous sports should be avoided.

There is no treatment which improves the prognosis, although symptoms, from heart failure or angina, can be alleviated. It is not amenable to surgical intervention. Drugs which increase myocardial contractility, such as digoxin and salbutamol, should be avoided. Those which reduce preload, such as nitrates, should be avoided or used with care. Beta-blockers, calcium antagonists and disopyramide are used but guidance from a cardiologist is needed.

4.6.3   AORTIC REGURGITATION

What is it?

The cusps of the aortic valve are damaged or distorted and fail to meet, closing the left ventricular outflow tract, during diastole.

What causes it?

It is caused by all the same processes which affect the valve in aortic valve stenosis and the two conditions commonly coexist, although one may predominate in its effects.

What happens?

(1)   Pure aortic regurgitation gives the left ventricle an increase in volume to pump, without any increase in pressure.

(2)   There is hypertrophy of the left ventricle with increase in muscle mass and chamber volume (dilatation) without any increase in the thickness of the wall.

(3)   Arrhythmias are common because of the dilatation of the ventricle.

(4)   Angina is a less obvious feature than in aortic stenosis.

(5)   The end result is left ventricular failure.

How do you know?

Routine medical examination may reveal a large left ventricle, collapsing pulse, aortic diastolic murmur and possibly concomitant aortic stenosis. Chest X-ray may show a large left ventricle.

Also:
- breathlessness, indicating left ventricular failure, may develop;
- a ventricular arrhythmia may cause palpitations, dizzy spells or syncope.

What do you find?

- Collapsing pulse with a large pulse pressure.
- Left ventricular impulse on palpating the precordium.
- A soft, blowing diastolic murmur over the middle of the sternum: best heard with the patient sitting in a chair, leaning forwards and breathing out.

What do you do?

The only treatment which provides anything except symptomatic relief is surgical valve replacement. Referral to a cardiologist for assessment should be arranged without waiting for serious symptoms to develop.

Long-term care is needed to:

monitor the progress of the disease;

supervise anti-coagulant therapy after surgery;

watch for complications of arrhythmias or heart failure.

Prevention of SBE is important as in aortic stenosis.

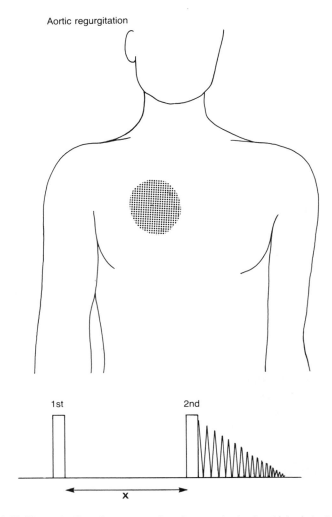

Figure 4.6F The early diastolic murmur of aortic regurgitation is a high pitched, blowing sound best heard with the diaphragm of the stethoscope with the patient leaning forward and holding breath out. It may also be heard at the apex

4.6.4 MITRAL STENOSIS

What is it?

Narrowing of the mitral valve area by fusion of the valve cusps resulting from rheumatic carditis in the past.

It is the commonest form of chronic rheumatic heart disease and it is still regularly discovered for the first time in patients who had rheumatic fever when young.

Who gets it?

Mitral stenosis occurs only in people who have had rheumatic carditis. Since rheumatic fever is often an insidious and undramatic condition and will have occurred many years before, it is common for the patient to give no history of it. In the UK, it is seen in the indigenous population over 40 and in immigrants.

What happens?

The mitral valve area is progressively reduced so that blood flow from the left atrium to the left ventricle is restricted.

The symptoms and signs will depend on the degree of stenosis and on the presence of other complicating conditions, such as mitral regurgitation, aortic stenosis, atrial fibrillation and hypertension.

Cardiac output is reduced, as the result of the overall reduction in blood flow through the heart. The left atrium becomes dilated and hypertrophied. Pulmonary venous pressure rises gradually, causing chronic pulmonary congestion and allowing time for compensatory mechanisms to come into play:

- lymphatic drainage from the lungs increases;
- pulmonary arteriolar tone increases, protecting the lungs from the full force of right ventricular output and causing an increase in pulmonary arterial pressure.

Pulmonary oedema eventually develops. There is hypertrophy of the right ventricle.

If right heart failure occurs, the pressure on the lungs is reduced and the patient is likely to feel better, despite the development of peripheral oedema.

How do you know?

Unlike aortic stenosis, the physical signs of asymptomatic mitral stenosis are not obvious and it is only rarely found as the result of a murmur being noticed on routine examination.

It is therefore usually diagnosed when symptoms occur.

The findings are:

(1)   Those due to raised pulmonary venous pressure (left heart failure):
  – breathlessness on exertion and on lying down;
  – paroxysmal nocturnal dyspnoea;
  – pulmonary venous congestion on chest X-ray.

(2)   Those due to low cardiac output:
  – fatigue;
  – poor peripheral perfusion: cold extremities.

(3)   Those due to atrial fibrillation:
  – at onset: sudden onset of heart failure, palpitations;
  – when established: emboli: systemic and pulmonary.

(4)   Those due to right heart failure:
  – peripheral oedema;
  – raised JVP;
  – hepatomegaly (with jaundice and cardiac cirrhosis in the late stages).

(5)   Those due to the structural changes in the heart:
  – enlarged left atrium on chest X-ray; P mitrale on ECG;
  – right ventricular hypertrophy on palpation of the cardiac impulse and on ECG;
  – opening snap and mitral diastolic murmur at the apex (Figure 4.6G).

(6)   Those due to associated conditions:
  – aortic valve disease occurs with mitral stenosis but it takes longer to develop and may be at an earlier stage;
  – hypertension.

What do you do?

Referral is not urgent because nothing sudden is likely to happen to a patient with mitral stenosis. However, assessment will be needed at some stage and anticoagulant therapy should be started immediately if atrial fibrillation develops.

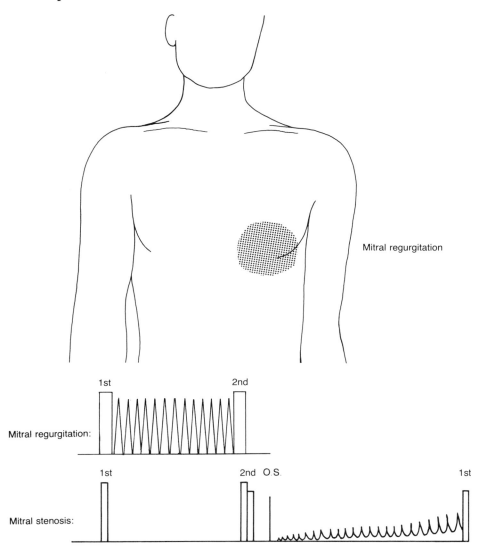

Figure 4.6G The pansystolic murmur of mitral regurgitation is best heard at the apex. It radiates into the axilla or towards the sternum. The mid-diastolic murmur of mitral stenosis is best heard with the bell of the stethoscope with the patient turned on the left side. It is localised to the apex

271

Fast atrial fibrillation is treated with digoxin and has to be carefully supervised. See Chapter 2.3 p.47.

There is a serious risk of SBE and the patient should be made aware of the risks and precautions needed and the medical records tagged to remind the doctors.

Surgical treatment is indicated in patients limited by symptoms. It need not be carried out prophylactically in asymptomatic patients as there is no increased risk of sudden death. It is not necessary for all patients with mitral stenosis, many of whom live in reasonable comfort with their diseased valve.

Long-term follow up is needed to:
- monitor the progress of the disease;
- watch for the development of aortic stenosis, hypertension or atrial fibrillation;
- supervise medication: digoxin and warfarin, once started, will be needed for the rest of the patient's life.

4.6.5 MITRAL REGURGITATION

What is it?

Diseased mitral valve cusps fail to close fully during systole so that blood regurgitates back into the left atrium when the left ventricle contracts.

What causes it?

Rheumatic heart disease: often accompanies mitral stenosis;
Ruptured chordae tendinae;
Floppy mitral valve;
Dilatation of the A – V ring in heart failure: the commonest cause.

What happens?

The left ventricle has to pump an increased volume and so undergoes hypertrophy and dilatation. The left atrium is exposed to increased pressure and becomes dilated and hypertrophied.

There is a rise in pulmonary venous pressure. If it is gradual, the effects on the lungs are similar to those seen in mitral stenosis.

Atrial fibrillation is common.

Thrombi may form on floppy valve cusps or in a fibrillating atrium and cause emboli.

Ventricular arrhythmias occur.
Both ventricles may fail (congestive failure).

How do you know?

Mitral regurgitation gives rise to a very loud murmur and so may be noticed at a routine medical examination.
The patient may complain of:
- fatigue and/or breathlessness due to left heart failure;
- peripheral oedema due to right heart failure;
- palpitations or acute symptoms of heart failure due to the sudden onset of rapid atrial fibrillation;
- symptoms related to embolic events.

What do you find?

- Signs of right, left or congestive heart failure (see Chapter 4.3 p.210);
- Atrial fibrillation;
- Signs of emboli;
- A large heart on clinical examination, with LVH and RVH on ECG and dilatation of both left atrium and left ventricle on chest X-ray;
- A loud pan-systolic murmur maximal at the apex but conducted all over the precordium (see Figure 4.6G p.271). The loudness of the murmur gives little indication of the severity of the disease.

What do you do?

Energetic treatment of heart failure and of atrial fibrillation is important.
Surgical valve replacement is useful in some people but is not appropriate if the condition is secondary to heart failure.
Prevention of SBE is important, as in mitral stenosis (see p.272).

4.7
Congenital Heart Disease

Who gets it?

Congenital heart disease affects about one child in every 130 live births. If a mother already has one affected child, the risk is trebled for the next pregnancy. It is more likely to occur in children with other congenital abnormalities, such as Down's syndrome. It is common complication of rubella in early pregnancy.

WHAT IS IT?

The development of the heart and circulation can be disrupted at any stage from conception to birth. The resulting range of possible abnormalities reflects the changes which occur during foetal life. They can be extremely complex: some, such as transposition of the great vessels, are incompatible with independent life; some, such as small VSDs, are insignificant. Some are correctible; some not. A complete description of all these is beyond the scope of this book. In this section, we discuss only those which are of most interest to family doctors.

They can be divided into three groups according to their haemodynamic effects.

Left-to-right shunts

At birth, the pressures on the two sides of the heart are similar, so little flow takes place if there is a communication between them. As the child's lungs develop, the pressures gradually assume the eventual differential. After that, any simple communication between the two halves of the circulation leads to a flow of blood from left to right because, at all points, the pressure on the left is higher than that on the right. The common ones are (see Figure 4.7A):

- Atrial septal defects (ASD)
- Ventricular septal defects (VSD)
- Persistent ductus arteriosus (PDA).

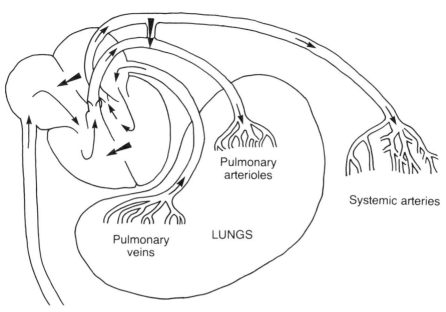

Figure 4.7A Left-to-right shunts

Right-to-left shunts

If the normal outflow from the right ventricle is impeded, for instance by pulmonary stenosis, the pressure on the right side of the heart may no longer be lower than on the left so that a septal defect then results in a flow of blood from right to left. This causes cyanosis and is known as cyanotic heart disease. It is typified by Fallot's tetralogy, in which a VSD and pulmonary stenosis coexist. (The other two elements of the misnamed tetralogy are an overriding, or dextroposed, aorta and hypertrophied right ventricle.)

Stenotic defects

These lead to a relative obstruction of the circulation, the results of which depend on the site of the defect and on its severity. The commonest are:
-   Aortic stenosis
-   Pulmonary stenosis
-   Coarctation of the aorta.

WHAT HAPPENS?

Attention is drawn to the presence of congenital heart disease in several ways:

(1)   Antenatal diagnosis by ultrasound scan:
- routine;
- screening of women at high risk, e.g. who have previously had an affected child.

(2)   Obvious distress at birth:
These will be referred immediately to a paediatrician.

(3)   Abnormality detected on routine examination:

Poor weight gain or delayed growth	Low cardiac output
Breathlessness	Hepatomegaly
Tachycardia	Cardiomegaly
Vomiting	Central cyanosis,
Murmur	squatting, clubbing.

Symptoms and signs appear at different times in different infants, depending on the type and severity of the lesion (Table 4.7A).

It is important that children are examined repeatedly, if significant abnormalities are not to be missed.

A suggested plan is for examinations to be carried out at the following intervals:

Birth	1 year
7–10 days	4–5 years
6–8 weeks	Adult.
6 months	

Table 4.7A Usual age of appearance of signs

At birth	Over 3 days	Over 3 years
Aortic stenosis	VSD	ASD
Pulmonary stenosis		PDA
		Coarctation

276

(4)   Feeding difficulty (due to breathlessness).

(5)   Failure to thrive during infancy or early years.

(6)   Repeated chest infections.

(7)   Cyanosis.

WHOM TO REFER?

Any sick child, in whom congenital heart disease is a possibility, should obviously be referred immediately. Difficulties arise in the case of well children with murmurs.

(1)   Stenotic lesions need early referral:
- murmurs from stenotic lesions are often present at birth, whereas those from shunts appear later.
- stenotic murmurs are unchanging and often loud.

(2)   Soft systolic murmurs at the left sternal edge are common:
- most are of no clinical significance, especially if variable, e.g. change with time, position and general condition, such as fever, excited, nervous;
- if in doubt, re-examine in a few weeks time.

(3)   A continous 'venous hum' below the clavicle may be confused with the machinery murmur of persistent ductus but the venous hum disappears with changes of position of the head. The machinery murmur of PDA does not appear until the child is 3 or 4 years old.

(4)   Certain lesions do not need treatment in childhood but cause serious problems later in life. These include mildly stenotic valves and shunts. There is a risk that patients who move, or who are lost to follow-up because they outgrow paediatric departments, will be overlooked. They should continue to have long-term follow-up from a cardiologist until formally discharged.

4.8

Bacterial Endocarditis

4.8.1 ACUTE BACTERIAL ENDOCARDITIS

What is it?

It is an infection of the endocardium covering the heart valves by virulent organisms. It can affect healthy valves.

Who gets it?

Apparently healthy people
Anyone with a severe infection or debilitating illness
Drug addicts using i.v. drugs
Diabetics
Immunosuppressed patients
Terminally ill patients.

What causes it?

It usually results from a bacteraemia or septicaemia in a debilitated or acutely ill individual.

How do you know?

The patient is acutely and severely ill.

What do you do?

Admission to hospital is necessary.

4.8.2 SUB-ACUTE BACTERIAL ENDOCARDITIS (SBE)

What is it?

It is an infection of the endocardium covering heart valves which are damaged by rheumatic carditis or congenital abnormality. It can also occur on prosthetic valves and other congenital cardiovascular abnormalities.

What causes it?

It results from a bacteraemia with an organism of low virulence, which would be insignificant in anyone without an underlying abnormality which renders them susceptible.

Organisms can enter the circulation during:
- dental procedures (especially scaling);
- endoscopy, especially GU procedures;
- surgical operations on the bowel;
- childbirth;
- intravenous injection by drug addicts.

Common organisms are: *Streptococcus viridans*, *Streptococcus aureus*, *Streptococcus faecalis*.

Uncommon organisms are: *Candida*, *Histoplasma*, *Rickettsia* (Q fever), *Chlamydia*.

Who gets it?

People with:
    abnormal valves: congenital or rheumatic
    prosthetic valve
    congenital lesions: persistent ductus arteriosus
                      ventricular septal defect
                      coarctation of the aorta.

What happens?

(1)   Vegetations, composed of bacteria and fibrin clot, form on the endocardial surface of the affected area.

(2)   The valve is progressively destroyed.

(3)   Pieces of the vegetations break off as infected emboli.

(4)   Low-grade septicaemia persists.

(5)   The mortality is high, even with treatment.

How do you know?

SBE may cause a large variety of insidious symptoms so that the diagnosis may not be immediately obvious. A high index of suspicion is needed in all patients at risk. The records should be marked so that the diagnosis is considered whenever they are seen. The patient should be advised to mention their underlying condition at every medical contact. They should not be given antibiotics without considering the possibility of SBE.

The main symptoms are:

Fever

Post-operative pyrexia

General malaise

Weight loss

'Fibrositis': myalgia, joint pains
or effusions

Mental disorders

Headache, meningism

Focal weakness, speech or
visual disturbance

Abdominal pain

Haematuria

Pneumonia

What do you find?

There may be no abnormal findings.
There may be:

Heart murmur (absent in 15%): may change

Low-grade fever

Anaemia

Clubbing

Embolic phenomena:

haematuria

subarachnoid haemorrhage

splinter haemorrhages (may be microscopic)

painful cherry red spots in finger tips (Osler's nodes)

neurological signs

Mental changes

Heart failure.

What do you do?

If there seems a serious likelihood of SBE, the patient should be admitted to hospital immediately.
   If there is real doubt, investigations may help:
   – FBC and ESR:
      normocytic anaemia
      WBC usually raised but may be normal or even depressed
      ESR raised;
   – Blood culture x 4: positive in 90% provided antibiotics have not been given.

Treatment must be carried out in hospital.

Prevention

This is an essential part of the management of patients known to be at risk of SBE (see above).
   Antiobiotic cover should be given for:
      All dental procedures
      Surgical operations
      GU procedures
      Endoscopy
      Biopsies
      Childbirth
      IUCD insertion: consider another method of contraception.

What regime?

– Amoxycillin:
   adults: 3 g, 1 hour before procedure
   children: under 10 years: 1500 mg
                     under 5 years: 750 mg.
– If allergic to penicillins, give erythromycin:
      1500 mg by mouth, 1–2 hours before procedure
      AND 500 mg, 6 hours later.

4.9

Cardiomyopathies

WHAT ARE THEY?

This is a group of diseases which affect heart muscle.

They are distinguished by different clinical pictures and by multiple causes.

WHAT HAPPENS?

Dilated cardiomyopathy

(1)   The heart muscle becomes weak and the heart dilated.
(2)   The A – V valve rings dilate and the valves become regurgitant.
(3)   Poor emptying allows the formation of thrombus and emboli.
(4)   Arrhythmias are common and may cause sudden death.

Hypertrophic obstructive cardiomyopathy (HOCM)

This is a familial disorder in which the myocardial fibrils are incorrectly arranged. It results in progressive thickening of the ventricular wall and obliteration of the lumen and obstruction to the outflow tract (aortic sub-valvar stenosis).

Restrictive cardiomypathy

Increased rigidity of the myocardium causes reduced compliance, which restricts ventricular filling.

Unless an underlying cause is identified and treated, all forms of cardiomyopathy are relentlessly progressive and are eventually fatal but the rate of progression is variable and may be very slow with long periods when little deterioration is apparent. Therefore, although the prognosis must be guarded, it need not be too gloomy.

WHAT CAUSES CARDIOMYOPATHIES?

Many causes have been described. Most are rare. The commonest to be met in everyday practice are those due to alcohol and thyroid disease, which cause the dilated form. Most of the rest are idiopathic; many are familial.

WHAT DO YOU FIND?

(1)   Symptoms and signs of:
        Heart failure
        Arrhythmias
        Angina
        Aortic stenosis.

(2)   ECG may show:
            LVH
            Non-specific S – T segment, T wave changes.

(3)   Chest X-ray: enlarged heart shadow.

WHAT ELSE MIGHT IT BE?

– Heart failure due to other causes, such as hypertension or ischaemic heart disease.

– Aortic valve stenosis.

WHAT DO YOU DO?

Patients, in whom a cardiomyopathy is suspected, should be referred to a cardiologist.
    While arranging this:

(1)   Treat underlying causes where possible:
        – alcohol abuse: it is impossible to be sure whether it is a contributory factor or not. If it is, very small amounts of alcohol can cause problems.
            Therefore, total abstention has to be advised in all patients with dilated cardiomyopathy;
        – thyroid disease: thyroid function tests should be performed on all patients with dilated cardiomyopathy.

(2)   Treat complications:
          arrhythmias
          heart failure.

WHAT TREATMENT?

This will be supervised by the cardiologist. Some patients benefit from beta-blockade. Some need other antiarrhythmic drugs. Digitalis should be avoided in HOCM unless there is atrial fibrillation. Heart transplant is a realistic option for some patients.

4.10
Pulmonary Embolism

WHAT IS IT?

The term is usually used to describe a clot of blood which enters the pulmonary arterial tree from elsewhere in the body. It can also be applied to fat or other substance.

WHAT CAUSES IT?

(1)   Thrombosis in the legs or pelvic veins or right atrium. No source is found clinically in 50%.

(2)   Predisposing factors are:
  − stasis:
        immobility
        postoperative: especially gynaecological
        air travel
        chronic illness, especially CCF;
  − obesity;
  − pregnancy and childbirth;
  − increasing age;
  − atrial fibrillation.

(3)   Septic embolus from infective endocarditis of the tricuspid valve is a rare cause, occuring mainly in drug addicts.

WHAT HAPPENS?

The effects are almost entirely haemodynamic and depend on the size of the embolus and the speed with which it breaks up into small fragments, which move into the peripheral arterial tree.

Large pulmonary embolism causes acute obstruction to the outflow from the right ventricle and right heart failure. The patient collapses with severe central chest pain and breathlessness, which may be difficult to distinguish from acute myocardial infarction (see Chapter 4.2 p.182). Death may occur very soon.

If the patient survives the initial shock, the clot may break up and be spread through the lung.

Small emboli cause infarction of lung tissue. There is less haemodynamic disturbance. The pain is pleuritic and localised to the area overlying the infarct. There may be bright haemoptysis. There is breathlessness, which seems disproportionate to the amount of lung affected, both at the time and for some time afterwards. A pleural rub may be heard.

WHAT DO YOU DO?

A small embolus may be the forerunner of a larger one and so the patient should be admitted to hospital for anti-coagulation, unless it is an expected terminal event. Anticoagulants are usually continued for about 6 months.

Prevention

(1)   Anticoagulation for:
          acute myocardial infarction;
          DVT; previous pulmonary embolism;
          atrial fibrillation;
          peri-operative for certain procedures.

(2)   Avoid immobility wherever possible.

(3)   Anti-thrombosis stockings in susceptible people.

4.11
Pregnancy

WHAT HAPPENS TO THE CARDIOVASCULAR SYSTEM DURING PREGNANCY?

Blood volume increases.
Peripheral resistance is reduced.
Stroke volume and heart rate increase.
Cardiac output increases: maximal at 28 weeks, returning to normal towards the end of pregnancy.
Blood pressure falls: lowest between 16 and 24 weeks.

These changes cause a number of symptoms, which are characteristic of normal pregnancy but which may mimic heart disease:
Breathlessness
Oedema of ankles (but JVP normal)
Tachycardia, extrasystoles, SVT
Collapsing (high-output) pulse
Systolic ejection (flow) murmur
Hypotension: postural or supine.

Heart disease in pregnancy is rare but it must be considered because it can be serious (12% of maternal deaths are associated with heart disease).

Pre-existing disease

Hypertension
Congenital heart disease
Rheumatic heart disease
SBE.

Disease resulting from pregnancy

Pulmonary embolism and cardiomyopathy of pregnancy usually occur during the puerperium.

HOW CAN PROBLEMS BE AVOIDED?

Pre-conceptual screening

Pre-conceptual screening is the ideal as it allows unhurried and full investigation of any abnormal finding, including X-rays, if needed.

It also allows identification of pre-existing physical signs, so that a murmur which appears later (during early pregnancy) will be immediately known to be physiological.

Ante-natal screening

A full examination of the cardiovascular system is an important part of the booking procedure.

Anyone with a diastolic murmur needs to be referred to a cardiologist.

Systolic murmurs cause the most difficulty.

(1)   Insignificant murmurs:
 – have not been heard previously;
 – are associated with a normally split second sound;
 – vary with position and on different occasions;
 – are associated with no ECG abnormality.

(2)   Significant murmurs:
 – have been noted before (e.g. in childhood);
 – may be associated with a fixed, split, second sound;
 – do not vary;
 – may be associated with ECG abnormality, e.g. right bundle branch block.

Significant murmurs should be referred.

Any symptoms or signs of heart failure are most likely to appear in the second and third trimesters.

4.12
Care of the Patient Dying of Heart Disease

Compared with the care of people dying of cancer, the care of the patient terminally ill with heart disease has received little attention.

This is strange because the problems are in many ways similar. Patients with severe, advanced heart disease suffer from fear of what will happen (of how they will die); grief at their loss of mobility, independence and imminent loss of life; difficulties in sharing the problems with those close to them, and difficulties of symptom control, often worse than those of the cancer patient. In addition to all this, it usually lasts much longer.

It is important that doctors and nurses caring for such people are aware of their needs and give them as much time, thought and attention as they can.

The problems can be considered in three groups, although they are related and interdependent:

Social
Emotional
Physical.

Social

This includes :
– Housing and domestic problems:
    Can the patient still manage stairs?
    Does he need a commode?
    Is there a telephone?
    Would a move be helpful, perhaps to sheltered housing?

– Who cares for the patient?
    Do they need help/relief/comfort?
    Can a break be arranged by admitting the patient to hospital or nursing home?

– Is financial help needed?
    Are they claiming all the allowances to which they are entitled?

Emotional

An opportunity to talk is most important. Fear and depression are serious problems and there is often difficulty in sharing them with relatives.

As with cancer sufferers, many patients find it difficult to accept that there is nothing more that can be done in the way of treatment. Most people deny the true situation, at least for a time, and insist that they are going to get better. The attendant professionals should not attempt to deceive patients with heart disease any more than they do those with cancer.

The doctor is not necessarily the best or only person to provide counselling. The clergy, social workers, psychiatric nurse and trained counsellors may be able to offer a different perspective.

Boredom aggravates depression. Occupation within the limitations of the disease is important.

Physical

Symptom control can be very difficult. The main problems are:
- those due to heart failure:
    breathlessness
    peripheral oedema
    fatigue; mental confusion;
- those due to angina;
- side-effects of medication (Table 4.12A).

Table 4.12A Side-effects of medication

Symptoms	Medication
Postural hypotension: dizziness, falls	Beta-blockers, calcium-channel blockers, ACE inhibitors, nitrates
Thirst/dry mouth	Diuretics
Headaches	Nitrates
Insomnia	Amiodarone
Muscular weakness; constipation	Diuretics (causing electrolyte disturbances)

The more energetically the heart failure and the angina are treated, the more of a problem side-effects become.

Nevertheless, small changes in medication can make a difference to the quality of life and it is worth juggling with different combinations and doses to find the best regime, even if it needs to be changed again after a time.

Sometimes a spell in hospital on maximum therapy can improve matters and allow the doses of the drugs to be reduced again, without an immediate relapse, when the patient goes home.

WHAT DRUGS?

The treatment is basically the same as that discussed in the other sections for the relevant underlying condition but some extra guidelines can be given here:

(1)　Patients dying from heart disease nearly always have some degree of heart failure:

- breathlessness at night is especially distressing and patients often sleep in a chair because they are afraid to go to bed and risk sliding down and becoming acutely breathless. The community nurse may be able to help with special pillows or even a cardiac bed.

- oedema may be severe, reaching to waist level and causing scrotal or vulval swelling and soreness. Severely oedematous parts weep and become infected. Again, nursing care makes a big difference.

- careful attention to diuresis is the mainstay of treatment: there is tremendous variability in the way in which patients respond. Some need massive doses of diuretics, while others are very sensitive to a modest amount. Different drugs suit different people. The only way to find out what suits the patient is to try it.

- the addition of an ACE inhibitor should be considered at an early stage.

(2)　Use the smallest effective dose of any drug.

(3)　A larger dose may be needed at first and can then be reduced when the symptom is controlled.

(4)　It is sometimes possible to reduce the dose of one drug by adding another with an overlapping effect: for instance, two different vasodilators. However, it has to be remembered that they may have shared side-effects. If GTN sublingual tablets cause headache, then it is likely that other nitrates, such as isosorbide mononitrate, or even nifedipine, will do so too.

(5)   Keep a constant watch for side-effects:

- old people may need very small doses of some drugs. The dose may have to be reduced as age and failing renal function render the patient increasingly sensitive.

- some drugs, such as digoxin, are cumulative and toxicity can develop with little warning in someone who has been on the same dose for years.

- urea and electrolytes should be checked at frequent intervals.

(6)   Both hypo- and hyperkalaemia are unpleasant as well as dangerous. It should be possible to avoid both:

- potassium is contained in fruit, including bananas, and vegetables;
- potassium-sparing diuretics can be combined with potassium-losing diuretics;
- potassium tablets are unpleasant to take and usually ineffective and unnecessary.

(7)   A small alcoholic drink at bedtime can make the patient feel more comfortable.

(8)   A very small dose of morphine or heroin by mouth can be helpful at night in a patient with intractable LHF: e.g. as tinct. opii: morphine 1% (10 mg/ml) or morphine or diamorphine elixir.

- DOSE: 2–5 mg of diamorphine or
           5–10 mg of morphine.

- It can be mixed with syrup, chloroform water or fruit flavouring, with or without alcohol.

BEREAVEMENT

Bereavement is just as hard to bear if the patient has died of heart disease as it is if the cause was cancer. In fact, sudden death causes particular feelings of shock and guilt and misery.

Families often fail to appreciate when a relative is likely to die and death comes as a surprise and a shock. This can be avoided if the doctor warns them that 'anything may happen'. If the patient then survives, they are pleased and relieved. If not, at least they are prepared.

The generally held belief that heart disease is linked with stress often has the effect of making relatives blame themselves for the death, although they may not admit it. It helps if the doctor tackles this problem and makes it clear that they are not to blame.

Physical symptoms are common in the recently bereaved and chest pain is frequently experienced by people who lose a relative from heart disease. It should be taken seriously, partly because they need reassurance but also because acute myocardial infarction commonly affects such people.

Long-term support may be necessary.

PART 5:

THE ROLE OF GENERAL PRACTICE

5.1
Introduction

This book is, to a great extent, concerned with diseases associated with coronary atheroma and hypertension. This is because these, of all cardio-vascular disease, form the most massive problem in western countries today and present doctors and all health care workers with the greatest challenge.

The challenge is to speed up the falling incidence of ischaemic heart disease by effective prevention and to improve the outlook for those with established disease by better diagnosis and management.

This is a massive task but it is clear that much could be done by an energetic multi-faceted programme of prevention and care.

Prevention is based on a recognition of risk factors; on early, accurate diagnosis and on appropriate use of available therapeutic tools.

None of these is the sole responsibility of the primary health care team but it has a major role, which we will try to expound.

There are two chapters in this part of *Commonsense Cardiology*:

Chapter 5.2: Risk Factors and Prevention;
Chapter 5.3: The Role of the Primary Health Care Team.

5.2
Risk Factors and Prevention

EPIDEMIOLOGY

Ischaemic heart disease accounts for 25% of the mortality and a high proportion of the morbidity in the adult population in the UK (Figure 5.2A).

In males between 45 and 60 years, 40% of all deaths are from ischaemic heart disease (Figure 5.2B, Table 5.2A). It is the main reason for men failing to reach retirement age. It is a major cause of early retirement and chronic disability.

An average GP will have five or six deaths from ischaemic heart disease, among his patients, every year. These will include three sudden deaths. He will also have to treat, help, support and comfort their widows and families. He is more likely to die himself from this cause than from any other.

Ischaemic heart disease is a much less common cause of death in Japan (about one tenth) and is rare in developing countries (Figure 5.2C).

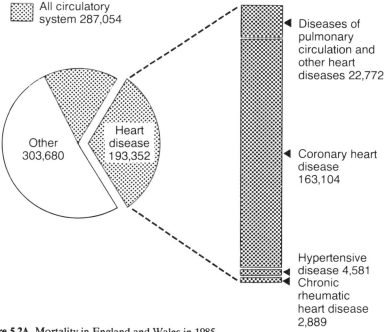

Figure 5.2A Mortality in England and Wales in 1985

297

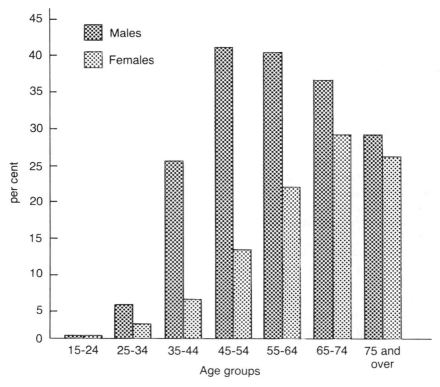

Figure 5.2B Deaths from coronary heart disease as a percentage of all deaths at selected ages, England and Wales, 1985

Table 5.2A Causes of death in England 1980

Causes of death	Numbers in England in 1980 (to nearest 1000)	Per GP with 2500 patients	Per District General Hospital serving 250 000 persons (to nearest 1000)
Ischaemic heart disease	145 000	5	500
Cerebrovascular disease	67 000	3	300
Cancers	60 000	3	300
Pneumonia	50 000	2	200
Bronchitis	18 000	1	100
Accidents	15 000	1 every 2 years	50
Suicide	4000	1 every 6 years	15
Total	544 000	20	2000

From Fry, J., Brooks, D. and McColl, I. (1984). *NHS Data Dook*, p.7. (Lancaster: MTP Press)

This is not a genetic predisposition. People who migrate from Japan and third world countries eventually assume the same mortality rate as their adopted country.

In the USA and Australia, mortality rates from ischaemic heart disease have been falling steadily during the last twenty years. In the UK, they remained steady until recently. They are now beginning to fall but only slowly (Figure 5.2D).

It is not clear why there are these differences. The problems are that the aetiology of ischaemic heart disease is multifactorial and that causal factors take a long time to manifest themselves. It is therefore inevitable that changes in a number of different factors will affect the incidence of the disease in the community and that alterations in lifestyle or treatment will take many years to have a measurable impact. For instance, although the incidence of the disease in Japan is low, it does appear to have been increasing during the last 30 years. It is hard to tell whether this is due to changes in diet, which are undoubtedly taking place, to the adoption of a more frenetic life style, to some other factor or to a combination of many things.

PREVENTION

"One half of all strokes and one quarter of deaths from coronary heart disease in people under 70 are preventable by the application of existing knowledge"

RCGP Report 1981

Prevention can only be based on a recognition of risk factors, early accurate diagnosis, better management of diagnosed cases, and an effective use of primary health care.

WHAT ARE THE RISK FACTORS?

These are factors which have been shown to have an association with an increased risk of heart disease above that expected for the population being studied.

The finding of an association does not automatically imply that measures to counter the factor will reduce the risk. This has been considered under the heading of hypertension but may apply to other things.

Male

Value	Country
425	N. Ireland (1985)
425	Scotland (1985)
406	Finland
400	Ireland, Eire (1983)
383	Czechoslovakia
354	New Zealand
354	England and Wales
349	Denmark
349	Sweden
333	Hungary (1985)
318	U.S.A. (1983)
315	Australia
302	Norway
290	Canada
255	West Germany (1985)
245	Netherlands
240	Israel
219	East Germany
178	Belgium
168	Italy (1981)
167	Poland
115	Spain (1980)
110	France
60	Japan (1985)

Age standardised death rate per 100,000 of standard population (European) Coronary (Ischaemic) Heart Disease - 1984 figures unless stated.

(Source: WHO statistics)

Female

Value	Country
212	Czechoslovakia
207	Scotland (1985)
204	N. Ireland (1985)
181	Ireland, Eire (1983)
171	New Zealand
168	Finland
168	Denmark
167	Hungary (1985)
164	U.S.A. (1983)
160	England and Wales
158	Sweden
156	Australia
150	Israel
143	Canada
119	Norway
112	West Germany (1985)
105	East Germany
102	Netherlands
81	Italy (1981)
77	Belgium
54	Poland
51	Spain (1980)
47	France
34	Japan (1985)

Age standardised death rate per 100,000 of standard population (European) Coronary (Ischaemic) Heart Disease - 1984 figures unless stated.

(Source: WHO statistics)

Figure 5.2C International incidence

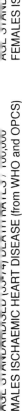

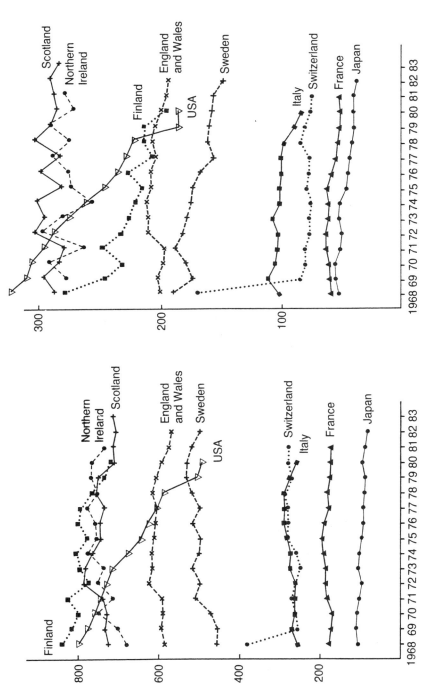

AGE STANDARDISED (35-74) DEATH RATES / 100,000
FEMALES ISCHAEMIC HEART DISEASE (from WHO and OPCS)

AGE STANDARDISED (35-74) DEATH RATES / 100,000
MALES ISCHAEMIC HEART DISEASE (from WHO and OPCS)

Figure 5.2D Comparative graphs

301

The known risk factors can be grouped under several headings.

Heredity

(1)   Genetic factors: family history of:
            IHD under 60 years.
            Hypertension
            Hyperlipidaemia
            Obesity.

(2)   Lifestyle factors (picked up in childhood):
            Unhealthy eating habits
            Smoking
            Obesity
            Alcohol abuse
            Attitudes to work; relationships.

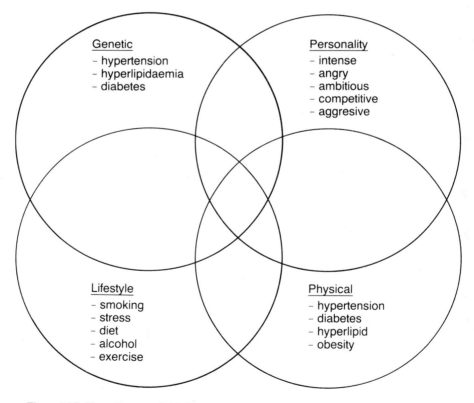

Figure 5.2E Venn diagram of risk factors

Lifestyle

Smoking
Behaviour (e.g. workaholic, competitive)
Relationships: marital, social, work
Diet: fats, sugar, salt, calories
Exercise: regular, long-term, aerobic exercise probably reduces risk.
    sudden, intense, anaerobic, competitive (e.g.squash) increases risk

Predisposing diseases

Hypertension
Diabetes
Hyperlipidaemia.

Personality type A

Obsessional
Rigid
Aggressive
Competitive.

Low social class or income

Figure 5.2F shows how social class relates to deaths from ischaemic heart disease.

REDUCTION OF RISK

The more and greater the risk factors operating in any individual, the more likely he is to develop ischaemic heart disease. They are synergistic and not simply additive so that having more than one risk factor multiplies the risk.

Not all the factors are equally important and their relative significance varies between individuals and races. However, some, such as smoking, obesity, diet and alcohol, can be altered and others, such as genetic and personality factors, cannot.

It is important to identify all the risk factors because the impact of those which cannot be altered may be lessened by reducing those which can. For instance, it is especially important for a smoker, with a bad family history, to give up and to have his blood pressure and lipids checked.

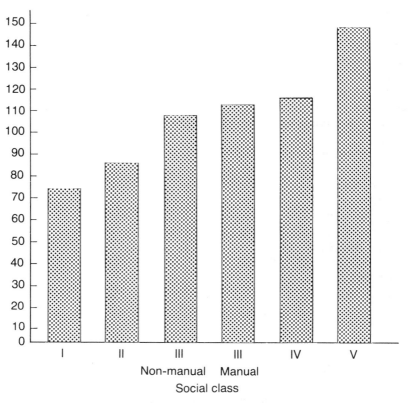

Figure 5.2F IHD incidence related to class [source: OPCS, 1986]

CAMEO

Joseph Parkin, 52, is a self-employed plumber. A short, stocky overweight man, he works hard, worries about VAT and smokes 20 cigarettes a day. His father died from a heart attack at 55 and he visits his doctor when he develops angina.

He is normotensive and his doctor treats him with a beta-blocker and nitrates and gives him all the usual good advice.

After 2 months he has made no progress. His total cholesterol is 6.8 mmol/l. His doctor then makes a further attempt to impress on him the importance of stopping smoking, losing weight and easing up on the work and worry. He arranges for him to see the surgery nurse once a week to help him with his diet and smoking.

He makes rapid progress and two years later is a slim non-smoker, symptom-free and needs no medication.

Table 5.2B Reduction of risk factors

Preventable (in children)	Modifiable (in adults)
Smoking	Smoking
Diet	Hyperlipidaemia
Obesity	Hypertension
Exercise	Diet
Alcohol abuse	Obesity
	Exercise
	Alcohol abuse
	Personality
	Compliance with treatment

The impact of risk factors can be reduced only if they can be identified and changes made. For any significant progress to be made, the problem has to be tackled from several directions, in a number of different ways and by many people.

Primary prevention

Primary prevention aims to stop disease developing. It encourages everyone to be a slim, happy, teetotal, non-smoker, eating a healthy diet, taking plenty of exercise, with an interesting and fulfilling occupation, no more stress than he can handle and satisfying, mature, family and social relationships. It would be expected to lead to the WHO definition of health:

"Health is a state of complete physical, mental and social well-being and not merely the absence of disease or infirmity."

This is unrealistically idealistic but remains a useful long-term aim. It involves making everyone conscious of health and their own responsibility for it without making them neurotic and fearful.

Secondary prevention

Secondary prevention aims to identify those with early (pre-symptomatic) disease and to reverse, halt or slow its progress. It implies screening of some sort. It implicitly includes all those matters included under primary prevention.

Tertiary prevention

This aims to limit the morbidity of established disease.

WHAT HAS TO HAPPEN?

The population has to be highly motivated and well-informed. Education and information has to be widely available in a variety of forms. Facilities for a healthy lifestyle should be available and accessible. Adverse factors such as smoking and food containing unhealthy ingredients should be actively discouraged. Facilities for screening for risk factors should be available and accessible. High standards of clinical care should be available.

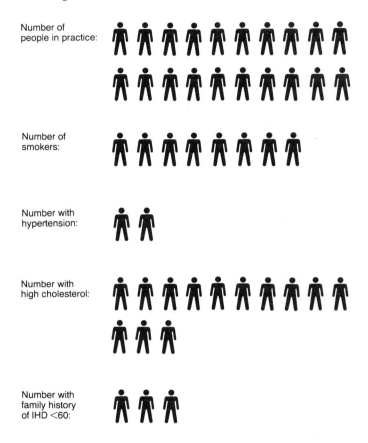

Figure 5.2G Incidence of risk factors in UK

WHO DOES WHAT?

A large number of people have to be involved if anything is to be achieved:
    Parents, teachers
    Journalists in every medium
    Food manufacturers, advertisers
    Cigarette manufacturers
    All health care workers and managers
    Politicians in both central and local government.

Possibly most important of all:
- Every individual, who, with the help of all the others, must take responsibility for his own health; lead a healthy life and be prepared to work in partnership with the professionals should his condition require it.

5.3
The Role of the Primary Health Care Team

A number of different agencies share responsibility for the prevention of cardiac disease (see Figure 5.3A).

WHAT CAN THE PRIMARY HEALTH CARE TEAM OFFER?

It has a number of major advantages, which at present are mostly under-valued and underused:

(1)   Accessibility: the members of the team are easily accessible to the population and the people are also accessible to the team.

(2)   Opportunity: 95% of all patients registered with a practice are seen at least once, by one or other member of the team, during any three-year period.

(3)   Staff and expertise (Figure 5.3B): all practices can, and most do, employ reception and secretarial staff; more and more are employing nurses, many of whom are willing and able to organise their own work in cooperation with other staff; in most practices, health authority-employed staff form an integral part of the team.

(4)   Familiarity and trust: the building and the staff are well known to the patients. Many have been familiar with them for many years, perhaps all their lives.

(5)   Knowledge and records of families are available over a long period.

All this means that information, education programmes and screening can be organised with little difficulty or expense and are likely to have the maximum effect. Long-term follow-up is readily accepted by the patient. Continuity of care is possible in a way that can never be achieved in a hospital outpatient clinic. Patients find the doctor approachable because he is familiar. They are therefore better able to express difficulties. Immediate access means that patients can discuss problems relating to treatment, instead of simply stopping it, if they suspect side-effects.

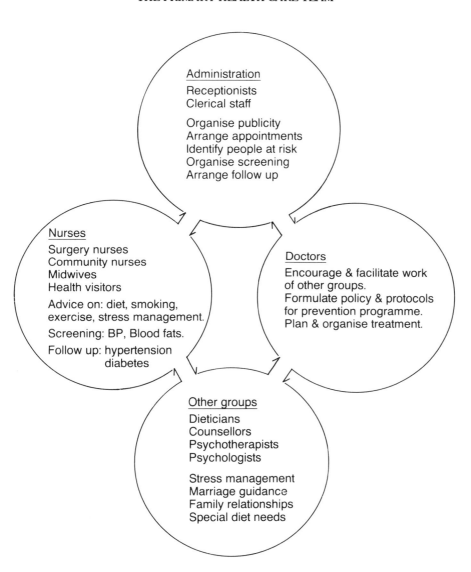

Figure 5.3A Groups involved in prevention

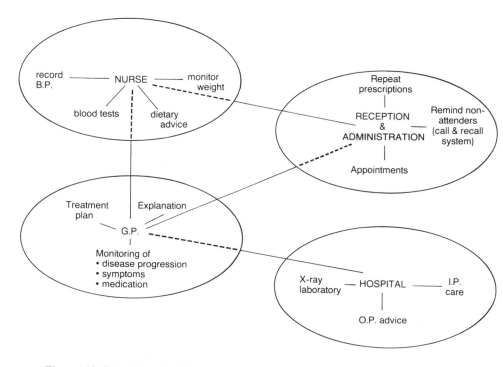

Figure 5.3B The primary health care team

WHAT ARE THE DIFFICULTIES?

There is no active tradition nor established system of prevention which can simply be continued. Anything which is done is done because someone in the practice has the interest, energy and enthusiasm to make it happen. This means that there is unlikely to be consistency of organisation or planning on either a national or a local scale, at least to begin with. Every practice has a different approach, ranging from making no provision of any sort for prevention through to a comprehensive education, screening and follow-up call and recall system.

This unevenness of service makes life very difficult for patients changing from one practice to another and for consultants working in local hospitals, who tend to gear their own provision to the lowest common denominator.

These problems are not insurmountable, as has been shown by the example of antenatal care which is shared, throughout the country, between hospital and general practice and where a very high standard is achieved.

HOW CAN IT BE SET UP?

Primary prevention

In many people, atheroma starts in childhood so prevention must start at, or before, birth. Total success is unlikely in the foreseeable future but it should be possible to delay the onset and to limit the extent and severity of the disease.

Ideally, prevention, in the form of health education, should be directed at the whole community. It is especially useful for GPs to be involved as their advice seems to have the most impact and is likely to be followed.

Preventive work should be concentrated on children and especially those with bad family histories.

Educational input from many sources can be used:
Antenatal classes
Mother-and-toddler groups
Playgroups
Schools
Colleges and universities
Media articles, broadcasts, campaigns and advertisements
Political pressure, e.g. to ban tobacco
Local leisure and sports facilities.

WHAT CAN BE DONE ABOUT WHICH RISK FACTORS?

Smoking

Smoking is by far the most important alterable factor. The evidence is clear, irrefutable and accepted by everyone.

What can be done about it?

(1)   Pre-conceptual counselling: women and their partners should be non-smokers before conception.

(2)   Antenatal advice: encourage/nag/bully/coerce/terrorise pregnant women to be non-smokers.

(3)   Passive smoking affects everyone: pregnant women and children should live in non-smoking households; all members of the household should be included in the anti-smoking campaign.

(4)   Help with giving up:
  – sympathy, support, suggestions, encouragement;
  – leaflets: see local health education officer;
  – frequent follow-up: e.g. during visits from health visitor, antenatal
     and baby clinic attendances, classes;
  – ask the patient to keep a chart of amount smoked and produce it
     whenever she is seen;
  – self-help group: the health visitor might help set it up; the practice
     provide a room for meetings;
  – posters and other promotional material from health education
     officer (see Figure 5.3C).

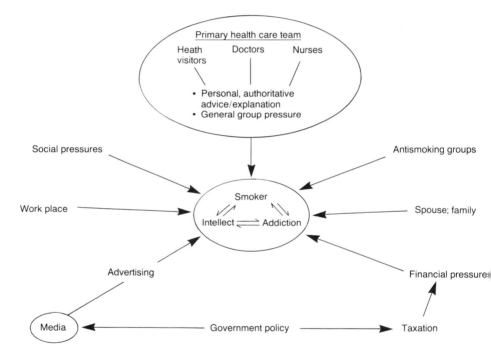

Figure 5.3C Help for smokers

Blood fats

Blood fats (see Chapter 4.2 p.144 for more on lipoproteins) are probably the
most important of all the risk factors.

A number of different factors influence the levels of fats in the blood and
the form in which they are carried:

(1)   Heredity: regardless of any other factor, some individuals appear to inherit a tendency to high triglyceride and LDL levels and thereby an increased risk of ischaemic heart disease.

(2)   Smoking and stress appear to have an adverse affect on the ratio of HDL to LDL cholesterol.

(3)   Exercise and relaxation have a beneficial effect on the ratio.

(4)   Sex: premenopausal women have a more favourable ratio than do men of the same age. After the menopause, women become more like men in this respect. This is at least part of the reason for the difference between the sexes in the age of onset of ischaemic heart disease.

(5)   Dietary fats: apart from its influence on obesity, diet plays an important part in the aetiology of ischaemic heart disease. This is almost entirely through its effect on the blood fats.

The proportion of energy derived from fat in the diet, in Britain, is 40%. A reduction to 30% would significantly reduce the incidence of IHD. In the USA, where this has been done, the average serum cholesterol has fallen by nearly 20% and the mortality due to IHD, by 30%.

It has also been shown that, in a group of healthy men aged 35–60, with serum cholesterol levels over 6.8 mmol/l, the effect of lowering this was to reduce the incidence of IHD events by 25% compared with controls.

A diet high in saturated fats (those found in dairy products and meat) causes an increased level of LDL. A diet low in saturated fats but high in polyunsaturated fats, is associated with lower levels of LDL. Fish oils have a protective effect. A high-fibre diet may reduce the absorption of fats.

A healthy diet

A healthy diet should contain:

(1)   Plenty of:
        Vegetables, including potatoes, rice, pulses
        Fruit, including bananas
        Cereals, including bread
        Fish of all kinds, but especially oily fish.

(2)   Moderate amounts (or none) of:
        Milk (skimmed for adults)
        Polyunsaturated fats, e.g. margarine

Lean meat, offal, poultry
Cheese (max. 8 oz per week full cream cheese like cheddar)
Eggs (max. three per week, including those in cooking)
Salt.

(3)   None of these:
Dairy fats: cream, butter, full cream milk
Crisps or chips (unless cooked in 'safe' oil, e.g. sunflower or corn oil)
Sausages, burgers, fat minced meat
Sugar or prepared foods with added sugar, e.g. most tinned fruit and
soups.

(4)   Only sunflower, maize or olive oil should be used in cooking.

Such a diet is suitable for everyone *over* the age of 5 years (it could cause
rickets if fed to infants).
It is important:
– to ensure that total calorie intake is adequate, especially in children,
adolescents and people doing heavy work.
– to check that smokers do not use the diet as an excuse to continue to
smoke: it is more important to give up smoking.

Patients with hyperlipidaemia need to adhere to the diet very strictly, should
omit eggs and cheese and may need medication as well (see Chapter 4.2
p.150).
For patient diet sheet, see p.327.

Exercise

Direct evidence of the beneficial effect of exercise is hard to find.
It probably:
– lowers the blood pressure in certain hypertensive individuals;
– improves the HDL:LDL ratio;
– promotes a feeling of well-being;
– lessens feelings of anxiety and stress;
– encourages non-smoking;
– helps to keep weight under control.

To have these effects, exercise has to be regular and reasonably strenuous.

Stress

Stress is probably important but this is hard to prove. What is important is not so much the amount of stress in someone's life, but his ability to handle it. Major life crises appear to be linked to an increased incidence of cardiovascular events; retirement and bereavement are especially important: death from a 'broken heart' is not a complete myth, although the mechanism is unclear.

People can be taught to improve their ability to handle stress (Figure 5.3D). Some companies organise schemes for this. Members of the primary health care team are well placed to identify people at risk from stress and to direct them towards help:

- relaxation classes
- behavioural psychologist
- psychotherapy
- counselling
- marriage guidance
- relaxation classes
- behavioural psychologist
- psychotherapy
- counselling
- marriage guidance
- child guidance.

Formal relaxation leads to a state of inactivity of body and mind, during which pulse rate, respiration rate and blood pressure fall and anxiety levels are reduced. It is not the same as sleep and some of the effects continue after the session is over. The beneficial effects are fairly well established but the activity has to be properly carried out. Lounging about in a negative, aimless way does not produce the same results, and, for some people, may even be stressful. The technique has to be taught: individually, in classes or groups, or using tape recordings.

Some people find formal relaxation very difficult and require frequent refresher courses or continuous instruction. These may be the people who need it most.

Obesity

People who are overweight are more likely to:

- Develop diabetes
- Have a high intake of saturated fats
- Have hyperlipidaemia
- Feed their children unhealthy diets

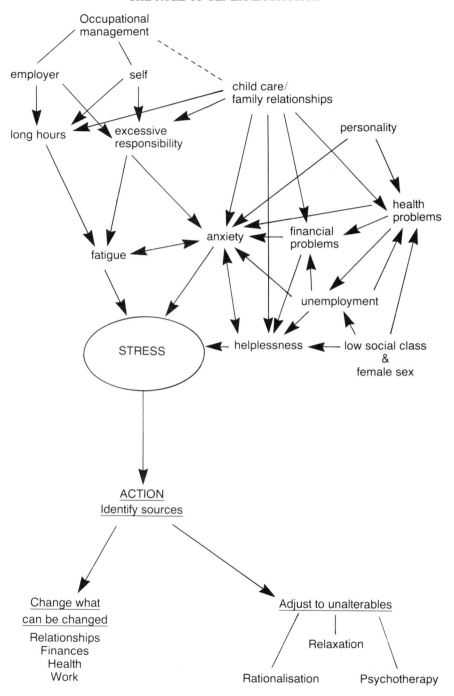

Figure 5.3D Stress management

- Develop atheroma, including ischaemic heart disease
- Be hypertensive
- Avoid exercise.

What can be done about it?

Most fat people find losing weight very difficult but all need to ingest fewer calories. All must understand that a lower calorie intake, i.e. a change in eating habits, has to be lifelong.

In theory, any reduction in calorie intake will cause loss of weight and it does not matter how it is done. But some people find some diets easier to follow than others, so a choice is important. Some can only lose weight when a diet is part of an overall fitness plan: thinking about nothing else, except what you may or may not eat, and when, may actually make eating less more difficult. Some prefer general guidelines which can be used by the whole family. Some need a rigid menu. Many find a high-fibre diet easier because it reduces problems with hunger and constipation. A slimming club or group may help.

SECONDARY PREVENTION

Anyone who:
  is a smoker
  is obese
  is hypertensive
  has a bad family history
  is diabetic
  has hyperlipidaemia
probably has a significant degree of coronary atheroma by the time they reach adulthood.

Secondary prevention can properly be directed towards identifying these risk factors and reducing them.

Where do you start?

Every adult's medical record should contain:
- a full history;
- a record of the BP at about 16 years of age, repeated every 5 years;
- a record of the serum cholesterol, measured at least once.

There is sometimes a delay before your previous medical record reaches your new doctor. It would assist him if you would provide a few basic details about yourself. Please would you complete this form as fully as you can and return it to the surgery.

FULL NAME .... DATE ....

FORMER SURNAME .... MARRIED/SINGLE .... DATE OF BIRTH ....

ADDRESS ....

.... POSTCODE ....

PREVIOUS ADDRESS ....

NAME & ADDRESS
OF PREVIOUS DR. ....

....

OCCUPATION ....

TELEPHONE NO: AT HOME .... AT WORK ....

FAMILY Please give details of the ages and states of health of the following
        relatives. If any have died, please give age and cause of death.

FATHER ....

MOTHER ....

BROTHERS/SISTERS ....

HUSBAND/WIFE ....

CHILDREN ....

PERSONAL DETAILS: HEIGHT .... WEIGHT ....

Brief details of any illnesses, accidents or operations (please continue overleaf
if necessary) ....

....

....

DO YOU SMOKE? .... HAVE YOU EVER SMOKED? ....

DO YOU SUFFER FROM ANY ALLERGIES? ....

HAVE YOU RECENTLY HAD A ROUTINE HEALTH CHECK/MEDICAL, e.g. AT WORK? ....

WOMEN ONLY

    DO YOU HAVE REGULAR PERIODS? .... IF NOT, WHEN DID THEY STOP? .

    DO YOU HAVE BLEEDING BETWEEN PERIODS? ....

    ARE YOU TAKING AN ORAL CONTRACEPTIVE? ....

    HAVE YOU HAD ANY PREGNANCIES? ....

    IF SO, PLEASE GIVE DETAILS INCLUDING
    DATES OF CONFINEMENT/MISCARRIAGE AND ....
    WEIGHT OF BABIES ....

    HAVE YOU HAD A CERVICAL SMEAR? .... IF SO, WHEN? ....

If you have any questions relating to this form, would you please discuss them
with the nurse at the surgery?

Figure 5.3E Registration form

318

If this is considered an impossible undertaking, then an attempt should be made to screen at least those at special risk, e.g. with bad family history, diabetes, recent bereavement (Figure 5.3E). These can be identified by asking everyone to complete a form on registering and by noting life events on patients already registered with the practice.

CAMEO

Joan Saltdean is 39. She has been an insulin-dependent diabetic since she was 15. Despite the best efforts of all the many medical personnel with whom she has had contact, she is hugely overweight and smokes heavily. She was admitted to hospital with an acute anterior infarct 2 months ago and has now had an angiogram, which shows peripheral coronary artery disease with no proximal stenoses, which might be amenable to surgery.

How can it be done?

(1)   Medical records must be well organised:
      A separate summary sheet for basic data is helpful (Figure 5.3F).
      If there is no summary sheet, it is difficult to keep track of who has been screened and of the results of those who have. Unnecessary repetition may result and borderline results, which need to be repeated, may be overlooked.
      Ideally, this should be done in a systematic way for all patients registered with the practice. Alternatively, it can be done opportunistically, when patients come to the surgery.

(2)   Opportunistic screening:
      In its simplest form, the doctor (or other member of the team) runs his eye down the summary sheet when the patient arrives and identifies any gaps in the record. Actual measurements (e.g. of BP) or gaps in the history may be completed by the doctor or by a nurse.
      Another method is for the receptionist to tag the notes to indicate which people have incomplete screening data before the session begins. The doctor is then immediately aware of the fact when the patient enters his consulting room. Alternatively, when the patient arrives, he or she can be invited to see the nurse first so that the gaps may be filled in.
      The most sophisticated systems produce a computer-printed appointments list for each doctor.

SUMMARY CARD

Recall date ☐☐☐☐☐☐   **MALE / FEMALE**

Name	
Address	
Date of Birth	SMWD Practice No.
Occupation and Spouse's Occupation	Doctor

Parity ☐   Rubella ☐

                              Polio ☐

Allergies   Tetanus ☐

                              Diptheria ☐

NOTES   Pertussis ☐

                              Measles ☐

Ideal Weight		Height	
Initial B.P.	1st	2nd	3rd

Alcohol	Date	Cytology	Weight	B.P.
Smoking				
Contraception				

Family History	M.I.	CVA	DM				
Father							
Mother							
Brothers							
Sisters							
Others							

Figure 5.3F Summary sheet

Opposite each patient's name is a list of the routine items missing or due to be repeated. The doctor may choose to ignore them if he is short of time or the patient is ill or reluctant. In this case, the list will reappear when the patient next attends. He may decide to complete some or all of the items himself or he may ask the nurse to do them. He may ask the patient to return on another occasion.

(3)   Selective screening:

- people at special risk are selected according to chosen criteria, e.g. age or family history;
- an age – sex register (paper or computer) is needed;
- can be carried out opportunistically, as above, or by sending special appointments;
- has the advantages of making sure that those most at risk are seen and that the screening does not delay the progress of a busy surgery;
- has the disadvantages of cost, of having to set up special sessions and of poor compliance. (Telephone appointments are usually cheaper and produce a better response than post but take time.)

CAMEO

Gary Johnson is 32 and has just moved to the area and registered with the practice. He completes the standard form which is given to all new patients. This reveals that his father died of a heart attack at the age of 54 and that he has not had his blood pressure taken.

He is sent a note offering him an appointment to see the nurse for a health check. His blood pressure is found to be 180/114 and his total cholesterol 7.4 mmol/l. He is advised to see the doctor for further management.

---

(4)   Screening at request of patients:

This happens, to some extent, already: few doctors refuse to take someone's blood pressure, if asked to do so. The main problem is that few people realise what should be done and those that do may not like to ask.

Publicity is therefore needed:
posters in the waiting room
leaflets
word of mouth: receptionists, nurses, health visitors
a regular practice newsletter

a practice booklet.

In these ways, people can be informed of what is advised and available and encouraged to take advantage of the service.

Which is best?

Every practice has to decide which approach suits it best. It is possible to combine elements of several different methods. Opportunistic screening of some sort is probably the easiest to set up.

CAMEO

Brian Major died suddenly 3 months ago from an acute myocardial infarct at the age of 48. He left a widow, Marion, and three children, Duncan, 12, Peter, 15, and Susan, 19. When he died, a note was made by the receptionist in charge of follow-up to consider screening the children in three months' time. Tags are put on their notes to remind the doctor who next sees them to discuss it. If they do not attend for a further 3 months, Marion will receive a letter.

All three children are found to be normotensive. Duncan and Susan have total cholesterol under 5 mmol/l. Peter has a total cholesterol of 7.2 mmol/l, which is then investigated further, treated and followed-up long-term.

What about other heart disease?

Secondary prevention can be directed against heart disease other than ischaemic heart disease:

- All babies should be examined at birth, at 6 weeks, at 6 months and at 4 years for evidence of congenital heart disease.

- Anyone with congenital or rheumatic heart disease should have this prominently recorded in his records so that antibiotic cover is given when needed and the risk of SBE always kept in mind.

- Coarctation of the aorta is difficult to detect in young children but the blood pressure is likely to be raised by the age of 16 years.

The DIY Medical Check-up

Why spend hundreds of pounds on a private medical check-up when you can do your own for nothing? Here is how:

- Have either of your parents or a brother or sister died from a stroke or heart attack before the age of 65 years?
  If yes, see the nurse for a check on the fats in your blood (free).

- Do you suffer from any of these symptoms?
  - Bleeding from the back passage.
  - Coughing blood.
  - Unexplained loss of weight.
  - Bleeding between periods.
  - Bleeding more than two years after the menopause.
  - Persistent indigestion or tummy pains.
  - Pains in the chest.
  If yes, then see your doctor (free).

- Are you overweight?
  If so, do something about it.
  If in doubt, strip and look at yourself from every angle in front of a long mirror (see nurse for weighing and diet sheet if you wish).

- Do you smoke?
  If so, **STOP**.

- Have you had the following health checks in the last five years?
  - Blood pressure.
  - Cervical smear.
  - Eye examination (over 40's).
  If not, make an appointment (free).

- Do you get regular exercise?
  If not, get going (not squash if you are over 40).

- Do you work excessively long hours and miss out on holidays?
  If so, re-organise yourself.

- Is your marriage creaking at the seams?
  If so, consider seeing a Marriage Guidance Counsellor before the seams burst open!

- Do you eat a healthy diet!
  Less sugar, dairy products and red meat than before (no pork or bacon): more fruit, vegetables, bread, cereals and fish.

MAKE THIS YOUR FITNESS YEAR

TERTIARY PREVENTION

This involves the careful follow-up and monitoring of patients with established disease to prevent avoidable morbidity. It can make a significant difference to the quality of life and in some cases to the mortality.

To have maximum effect, it has to be formally organised. It is not enough to leave it to the patient to seek help as and when he thinks he needs it. Many early warning signs do not produce symptoms and the patient may attach little significance to symptoms which are in fact important. No one can be forced to have medical check-ups, but people who need them should be encouraged to do so. At least doctors should inform patients of what current practice is, so that they can decide whether to accept it. Most do and feel comforted and reassured that they are being cared for.

Some sort of recall system is needed to identify those who fail to attend regularly.

How can a recall system be organised?

(1)   Card index:
   –   divided into 12 sections: one for each month;
   –   card is removed when a patient is seen and a further date arranged, and placed in the section for the month in which his next appointment falls;
   –   any cards remaining in a section at the end of the month are those of patients who have failed to attend. They can be reminded by telephone or post;
   –   No doctor time is involved.

(2)   punched cards: sorted manually in a similar way to the card index.

(3)   computer systems: these are simply an automated form of the card index.

Shared care

In theory, it should be possible to arrange for patients suffering from cardiovascular disease a system of shared care similar to that now universally adopted for antenatal patients. It works extremely well in the obstetric field to the benefit of all concerned. There is no reason at all why the same principle should not be applied to the care of everyone who needs input from both consultant and family doctor. It would be especially appropriate for people with heart disease.

A co-operation card (Figure 5.3G), similar to that carried by pregnant women, would enable doctors to keep in touch and save writing letters except in the most complicated cases.

How would it work?

(1)   Most routine care would be carried out by the family doctor. He or she would give:
   - support and encouragement;
   - advice about lifestyle: smoking, diet, exercise, sex, attitudes to work, marriage, children etc;
   - liason with employer;
   - support and advice for family.

Outside	Back		Front	
Name of GP:	Dr P. L. Endsleigh		Name:	Jeremiah CAMPBELL
Address:	The Health Centre Main Street Tumbletrees		Address:	73 Mansfield Drive Tumbletrees Wendshire
Tel. no:	7321-43670		Tel. no:	7321-56973
			D.O.B.	22 June 1927
			NHS No: SYP 236.7	Hosp No: 220627
Name of Consultant:	Dr R. S. Spindle		Diagnosis:	Coronary artery disease Angina
Hospital:	Tumbletrees General	FOLD	Allergies:	none
Tel no:	7321-57236		Next of kin:	Mrs Susan Campbell wife s/a

Inside				
Date	Problems	Observations	Drugs	Next appt.
?.9.88	Angina sl. better SOB on exertion Working F/T	P.76 reg. 158/94 JVP↓ No oedema Heart unchanged	Atenolol 50 mg once daily ISMN 20 mg twice daily GTN spray prn	1 year

Figure 5.3G Shared care card

(2)   Prescribing: to be safe, this really needs to be done by one person with access to all the information about the patient. This can only be the family doctor who is responsible for identification of new symptoms and side-effects of drugs. Disastrous problems can arise from a system where different consultants (or junior doctors), in different departments, even in different hospitals, all prescribe for one patient without each knowing what the others are doing.

(3)   Routine visits to the hospital: these would be at very long intervals for most patients and for many they would be completely unnecessary.
       For some, the visits would be supplemented or replaced by a postal report from the family doctor or the patient himself.
       When the patient did attend the hospital, he would always be seen by the consultant or registrar.
       Extra appointments would be easy to arrange at short notice, if the GP needed help or advice.

This would all be made possible because the numbers of patients attending the outpatient clinic would be reduced.

What are the advantages of shared care?

Under the present system, many important aspects of tertiary prevention are neglected. Patients are often seen in outpatient clinics by junior doctors, who do not know them and who are too inexperienced and too hurried to do the job properly. It is not even a particularly useful learning experience for them and few enjoy it. They stay such a short time in each post that no patient is likely ever to see the same doctor more than once. It is impossible to incorporate trust, confidence or continuity into such a system.
    This is unavoidable when such large numbers of people attend for follow-up over extended periods of time.
    Because the GP sees the patient as having been 'taken over' by the hospital, he sees no role for himself and leaves it all to 'them'. The GP's interest and expertise shrivels. With shared care, it revives and expands.

Can it be done?

It is certainly possible but it needs enthusiasm, mutual trust and co-operation, which are not yet available everywhere.

Healthy Diet: For adults and children over 5 years

Aim

To provide food of sufficient quality and content to:
– keep your weight steady and correct
– enable you to feel fit, well and active
– to keep you free from disease

Quantity

Eat as much as you feel you need. If you are underweight, eat more and at shorter intervals, e.g. frequent snacks. If you are overweight, eat less: choose filling, low-calorie foods. Do not miss meals.

Content

Eat plenty of these:
– Fruit of all kinds, including bananas
– Vegetables of all kinds, especially potatoes, beans, peas and rice
– Wholemeal bread and cereals
– Fish
– Poultry.

Eat moderate amounts of these:
– Lean meat
– Skimmed milk
– Margarine high in polyunsaturated fats
– Low-fat cheeses: cottage cheese, some Dutch cheeses.

Eat very little of these:
– Eggs: maximum three a week, including those in cooking
– Whole-milk cheeses, e.g. cheddar
– Foods containing sugar or fats or both: watch tinned fruit, soups, sausages, burgers, cakes, biscuits, cereals
– Salt.

Eat none of these:
– Fat meat, sausages, bacon, beefburgers, pork
– Cream cheeses
– Cream
– Butter
– Whole milk
– Potato crisps
– Sugar
– Fruit squashes, jams, sweets, chocolates, ice cream.

Use sunflower, maize or olive oil for cooking.

Books for Further Reading

For doctors

British National Formulary (London: British Medical Association and The Pharmaceutical Society of Great Britain)

Coronary Heart Disease, the Need for Action (London: Office of Health Economics)

Factfile leaflet series (British Heart Foundation)

Beevers, D.G. and MacGregor, G.H. (1987). *Hypertension in Practice*. (London: Martin Dunitz)

Guyton, A.C. (1987). *Human Physiology and Mechanisms of Disease*, 4th Edn. (W.B. Saunders)

Opie, L.H. (ed.) (1987). *Drugs for the Heart* (Grune and Stratton; Harcourt Brace Johanovitch)

Oram, S. (1988). *Clinical Heart Disease* (London: William Heinemann)

ECGs:

Hampton, J.R. (1980). *The ECG Made Easy*, 2nd Edn. (Churchill Livingstone)

Hampton, J.R. (1986). *The ECG in Practice*. (Churchill Livingstone)

Rowlands, D.J. (1982). *Understanding the Electrocardiogram: A New Approach.* (ICI)

Watson, H. (1984). *Disorders of Cardiac Rate, Rhythm and Conduction.* (Beaconsfield Publishers)

For patients

Heart Research Series (British Heart Foundation)

Index